Special Care

Special Care

Medical Decisions
at the Beginning of Life

Fred M. Frohock

The University of Chicago Press
Chicago and London

Fred M. Frohock is professor of political science in the Maxwell School of Citizenship and Public Affairs, Syracuse University. He is the author of *The Nature of Political Inquiry* (1967); *Normative Political Theory* (1974); *Public Policy: Scope and Logic* (1979); and *Abortion: A Case Study in Law and Morals* (1983).

95 94 93 92 91 90 89 88 87 86   5 4 3 2 1

Library of Congress Cataloging in Publication Data
Frohock, Fred M.
  Special care.

  Bibliography; p.
  Includes index.
  1. Neonatal intensive care—Decision making.
2. Neonatal intensive care—Moral and ethical aspects.
3. Neonatal intensive care—Economic aspects.
4. Neonatal intensive care—Social aspects. I. Title.
[DNLM: 1. Critical Care—in infancy & childhood.
2. Decision Making.   3. Ethics, Medical.   4. Intensive
Care Units, Neonatal. 5. Neonatology. WS 420 F928s]
RJ253.5.F76   1986   362.1'9892'01   85-31806
ISBN 0-226-26581-1

Contents

Introduction

Neonatology as currently practiced has raised a number of moral and rational problems. Like most professions, this branch of medicine aims at securing discrete goods, is composed of individuals skilled in securing these goods, and is supervised by those who are experts within the practice. Yet precisely the effective exercise of complex skills to secure desirable goods—health, life—has produced outcomes that are controversial. A variety of physical conditions that would have been fatal a decade or more ago are now treated, with the result that some individuals survive at levels of life so low as to raise questions about the usefulness of therapy in such cases.

The range of physical problems now treated in tertiary care neonatal units is impressive. Infants who are born prematurely at twenty-four weeks and weigh less than five hundred grams now can pass thresholds that warrant aggressive therapy. Infants who were routinely passed over for treatment a short time ago—those who suffer from severe necrotizing enterocolitis, spina bifida, hyaline membrane disease, even hypoplastic left heart—are now candidates for therapy. In some cases, perhaps many, the results are good. Infants survive to lead fulfilling lives. But a growing number of patients survive only to be tethered to life-support mechanisms, unconscious or suffering from unremitting pain for years and sometimes for the duration of their lives. No other fallacy of composition has a harder bite: rational and moral practitioners who secure desirable goods find that *because* they are so skilled the outcomes of their practice cast doubt on whether they should be doing what they do so well.

The problems addressed by neonatologists occur infrequently. Babies born at twenty-seven weeks gestation or earlier amount to only 0.05 percent of all live births. Genetic disorders of any sort are found in less than 5 percent of live births. Chromosomal problems are even less frequent, occurring in fewer than 0.5 percent of live births. And not all premature babies, or babies with genetic or chromosomal disorders, even require intensive care. But when the low frequencies of problems from prematurity and genetic or chromosomal abnormalities are combined with the percentages of babies needing intensive care for severe infections (like beta strep) and for other problems, and when these data are extended across the United States, they translate into impressive totals. Approximately 250,000 babies (out of 3.5 million born) receive intensive care in the United States each year. One irony is that the skills of neonatologists in treating prematurity and birth abnormalities have created additional demand for pediatric therapy. The most common problems in pediatric medicine today are the illnesses and deficiencies caused by premature birth. Many of these premature babies would not have lived to reach pediatrics a decade or more ago. Hospitals also report that between 20 and 30 percent of their pediatric admissions are due to genetic abnormalities. These admissions are largely attributable to the growing success of neonatologists in keeping babies alive who have serious genetic disorders.

The decisions made by neonatology staffs are among the hardest in medicine. The patients in neonatology are at the beginnings of life. Successful treatment can mean sixty to seventy years or more of life for the individual who recovers. No other type of medicine has a higher payoff for overcoming illness. But the downslope is equally steep. A patient who does not survive loses all of that life. Even worse is another type of failure: the staffs at neonatology nurseries are haunted by the infants who survive without enough physical resources to recognize anyone or anything. Such children are the products of prodigious medical skills. And they remind both doctors and nurses of the limits and paradoxes of effective medical care.

Neonatal staffs must sometimes decide whether to treat infants at all and, once treatment has begun, whether and how to end therapy if the treatment has not succeeded. The thinking that goes into these decisions is at once ambitious and halting. Physicians must assess the physical conditions of infants who cannot talk, or complain, or even know what troubles them. The level of skill required for diagnosis in such conditions is exceedingly high. Physicians must also consult with parents and arrive at decisions jointly supported by medical expertise and parental wishes. They are also aware of the law and sensitive to the possibility that legal authorities may find some therapy decisions interesting. The decisions made in such

circumstances are a curious amalgam. The doctor-as-authority competes with the doctor-as-pragmatist. Physicians and parents combine different perspectives on a single team. When the team falls
apart, decisions on treatment are the result of (often protracted)
negotiations between doctor and parents. The image of the doctor
as solitary authority on treatment is almost never realized in neonatology nurseries.

I gathered the empirical data for this study during four months of
participant observation at a neonatal intensive care nursery. The
"participant" activity was of course passive. I did not help the staff
in treatment but merely observed from close up what was happening. My access to the nursery was virtually complete and I took
advantage of it. At times it seemed that I spent more time in the
nursery than at my home. The staff, with very few exceptions, was
willing to talk to me at length. Twenty-seven taped interviews and
numerous other interviews not taped, over twenty notebooks, and
a logbook recording my reflections constitute the empirical materials of the study. I have added to these materials some discussions
of current issues to place these experiences in a more global perspective. A third set of materials—the philosophical treatment of the
issues in neonatology—helps fill in what I mean by a global view.

Anyone who spends time in a neonatology nursery will see
things he has never seen before. My experiences were so interesting
(by turns intense and routine) that I want to communicate them to
the reader as I lived them. Using the chronological entries in the
notebooks seems the most effective way to do this. Doctors say that
those outside medicine, by which they mean academics and
lawyers, do not understand what medicine is really about. Presenting the material in the way I do here is a way of admitting that they
are right. I hope the reader will be able to absorb the nursery
experience as it is known by participants.

The goals of the study should be clear from a reading of the work.
I want to describe a social practice that, by its logic, employs both
technical and moral languages. Physicians are applying complex
medical knowledge that unavoidably relies on ethical terms like
rights, interests, consent. The contextual forces affecting rationality
have been explored in the social sciences in a much more detailed
way than have the effects of context on moral principles. Yet moral
principles are no less affected by the social practices that they
invade. Since there is no reason to think that the languages of
different discourses evolve in uniform ways, recent changes in

medical care should create inconsistencies between the languages of medicine and morality. My own conviction, stated and elaborated later in the book, is that rights languages are the main casualties of changes in medical technologies. But the conviction will not be communicated effectively unless the demonstration succeeds. The reader is asked to listen to the participants as they employ a grammar and even a script drawn from earlier human experiences that do not resemble the events they are currently confronting.

The conclusions of the study will be slowly formed throughout the work, in discursive form until the last chapter (where they are stated, I hope, with some clarity, tightness, and force). The discussion that is shortly to begin will address (a) the types of decision made in therapy, (b) the languages appropriate for these decisions (especially rights versus harm language), and (c) the institutional forms which are compatible with rational therapy decisions. I will argue in the course of the work that therapy decisions in hard cases may always be discretionary, though constraints can limit this natural latitude in decisions; that rights neither clarify nor effectively constrain therapy decisions; that the use of a harm principle may be a better guide than rights in rational decisions on behalf of infants in neonatal nurseries; and that, as a consequence of rational requirements in therapy, the legal system is inept as an instrument to make or oversee therapy decisions. The view set out here is empirical (at the start) and normative (at the end)—a conjoining of styles and theories objectionable, I would think, only to the most primitive of positivists among us.

The entire study is influenced by the anomalous relations between moral languages and the events of neonatology. Arthur Adkins, in *Merit and Responsibility* (Chicago: University of Chicago Press, 1960), has described the ways in which Plato reassigned Homeric notions of virtue to the city-state. Terms used exclusively to refer to individuals or families, and which described heroic actions, were assimilated to justice and used to refer to the "quieter virtues" of social cooperation. New conditions, in this case the development of political societies, led to a reconstruction of language to accommodate these different social realities. I argue that contemporary moral terms like *rights* are inappropriate in a neonatal nursery. The new and, in many cases, unique medical events require a different moral vocabulary. The introduction of *harm* in place of *rights* is a reconstruction of the language of medical staffs. But the reconstruction is drawn from a vocabulary of medicine found in the

Hippocratic oath, and so is more deeply entrenched in medicine than is *rights* language.

Moral language is often demarcated from empirical language as groups become polarized over events. Homeric societies may have been inclined to view virtue as an empirical term, so settled were its sense and reference. But justice was a source of evaluative dispute to the Sophists, who discussed the concept in different and more divisive circumstances (where standards were confused or ambivalent). Debates today over the sanctity of life, the meaning of human being or person, rights to life and treatment, are not simply disputations over facts or words. They are political disputes in which the participants have appropriated evaluative languages that reflect their goals. It is impossible in such circumstances to suppose that a work like this one can be a cool and neutral study. The reconstruction of language offered here is unavoidably a partisan undertaking that favors some political values over others. But the language of harm recognized here has one advantage over rival vocabularies. It is an instrument found within current medical practice that can accommodate the new realities of neonatology.

Let me add that the interview material I use to provide the views of actors in this study is drawn from taped interviews. Not all of the interviews I recorded have been introduced in the text, nor is any one interview reproduced in its entirety. I have tried to select those sections from the interviews that most effectively set out the thoughts I heard expressed frequently and strongly in my study of the neonatal nursery. Except for very light editing (for grammatical purposes only), the interview material is a direct transcription from the tapes.

Everyone has a story to tell in this work. We are, as they say, the apes who dream while awake. These dreams, when ordered and mediated by reality, can be the instruments that disclose the truths of our experiences. To see the truths of the special care nursery requires that the voices of the participants be heard extensively and that the ordinary life of the nursery be communicated in detail. The epistemology informing this exercise is well known. If it could be stated in a brief phrase, I would choose the expected words: understanding is found in action, not in contemplation. That the action in this case is vicariously experienced by the reader will not, I hope, compromise the ambitions of the project.

All of the names used here—hospitals, individuals—are fictitious, with two exceptions. My name is actually Fred Frohock and I have a younger daughter named Christina. The events, without exceptions, are recorded as they happened. They are all real, though their reality as events in the world is obviously different from their reality in the discourse here. I am grateful to many participants for helping me see these events. Unfortunately I cannot name most of them without jeopardizing the confidentiality pledges I have made. Two of the most helpful individuals can be thanked publicly, however. Dr. Robert Daly helped me gain initial entrée to the neonatal nursery and read my early research proposals and papers on this study. His advice and comments have been very helpful. Dr. Henry Sondheimer was my main connection to the nursery. He opened doors for me, helped get me back in the nursery after I was expelled in the early going, and was a constant and useful source of information. He also read the entire first draft of the book and helped me avoid any number of technical errors. I am also grateful to Dr. Albert Tripodi for helpful comments and to my research assistant, Kent Rissmiller, who did most of the library work in putting together the bibliography. My wife, Val, and older daughter, Renée, provided just the right amounts of emotional support during the intensive participant-observation months. And I am especially happy to thank my younger daughter, Christina, who created most of the fictional names used in the book and who jolted me into doing a work like this with her casual but stinging comment some time back—"The problem is, Dad, your books read like reference books."

I wrote the first draft of the book while being supported by a Syracuse University Senate Research summer grant, funds provided by BSRG Grant 507 RR077068-19, awarded by the Biomedical Research Support Grant Program, Division of Research Resources, National Institutes of Health. Additional money to transcribe the interview tapes was provided by Guthrie Birkhead, dean of the Maxwell School. I discussed some of the early ideas in the book at one of our bi-monthly meetings of the Center for the Study of Citizenship. The core group of the Center consists of nine Syracuse faculty from various disciplines. I am pleased to be a member of this group and record my thanks for an excellent discussion of the Center paper that preceded this book. It was at that meeting, for example, that I shifted my thinking from utilitarian to classical notions of *harm*.

Because I have agreed to mask the identities of parents and staff, I must thank these two groups collectively. I am grateful to the parents for sharing with me their thoughts and feelings on what was for most of them the most trying experience of their life. The neonatal staff at the hospital was, and is, excellent. My time in the hospital was one of the most interesting experiences of my life, in large part because of the doctors and nurses in the intensive care nursery. But it is to the patients, who can reach out and touch emotions you never knew you had, that I dedicate this work. I will never forget one of them.

FRED M. FROHOCK

1
The Nursery

1

It is a windless January 26. The skies are light gray, heavy with snow that will probably fall late in the afternoon. Inside the neonatal nursery at Northeastern General Hospital are thirty-four very young babies. Some are sleeping. Others are awake with an alertness that masks their illnesses. Still others are between sleep and wakefulness, their brains and nervous systems operating at only a fraction of the capacity of normal babies. These are the infants who will never know the world they live in. They are in a permanent vegetative state. Some of the other babies in the nursery have happier prospects; they are transients. These babies will recover quickly and permanently. Their stay in the hospital will be only a dim memory to their parents as they grow normally into adults. Other babies will never leave the hospital. Some will die in the nursery; others will be transferred upstairs to Pediatrics, where they will die. At this moment all of the babies in the nursery are being treated and stimulated by the nursing staff. It is one o'clock in the afternoon, one of three times during the day that staff members go through set routines of infant care.

The neonatal nursery at Northeastern is a tertiary care center (the most advanced type of care) with a reputation for careful and skilled treatment of babies. It has been a part of the hospital for only seven years, its own recent origins marking the newness of neonatology as a medical specialty. As recently as the early 1970s infants born prematurely, or with severe birth defects, were treated by the hospital's regular pediatricians in the obstetrics ward or in general-use intensive care facilities. Now such infants are immediately transferred from the obstetrics ward, or transported by ambulance or helicopter if born in one of the regional hospitals serviced by Northeastern, to the special neonatal nursery. There a battery of technological devices and therapies keeps infants alive who would formerly have died quickly and without fanfare.

The first impression one has of the neonatal nursery is that it is a very *busy* place. It contains forty beds in two wings. One wing (level one) contains the most critically ill infants. The other wing (level two), tranquil by comparison, has babies who are less critical (though still seriously ill by any medical standards). Both wings are usually filled, often crowded beyond capacity, with babies. Numerous people move in and out of the corridors and rooms. One hundred and seven nurses are assigned to the nursery, though only about sixteen to eighteen are on duty on each shift. The nurses see the babies continually when working. There are in addition both physicians and medical students on regular duty in the nursery: four staff neonatologists, three Fellows (pediatricians in two-to-three-year training to be neonatologists), three residents (in their second and third year of general pediatric training), three pediatric interns, and two fourth-year medical students. The nursery is also populated with casual visitors: respiratory therapists, lab technicians, lab specialists for more elaborate tests on the babies, X-ray technicians who appear with mobile X-ray units that issue warning noises I associate with large pieces of construction equipment on the move, doctors from other specialties who make rounds (cardiologists, orthopedists, dermatologists, etc.), anesthesiologists who appear for special assignments, respiratory students from the local community college appearing in groups two or three times a week, social workers, physical therapists (who write pithy notes to the nurses on the proper positioning of the babies), medical students on tour of the facility, cleaning staff, and—finally—the families of the babies, who have twenty-four-hour access to the nursery and who bring to the unit some of the intense human emotions found in the hospital. It is a dense and active place, at times like a Bosch painting in movement.

On this particular afternoon Dr. Catherine Richmond, the head of the nursery, is guiding me slowly through both wings, though we stay only in the halls during this first visit. The nursery is on the fourth floor of the hospital, accessible by stairs or elevators. Each wing is separated by a main hall. Within each wing another hall separates suites of rooms. To go into the rooms where the babies are located requires washing up and donning a clean gown. Richmond and I slowly tour the halls in our street clothes, peering in at the babies through glass windows. As we walk, Richmond comments on several of the babies and talks about the way the nursery works.

She stresses, as do other doctors I talk to later, the scarcity of medical resources. Scarcity occurs at both the macro and micro levels in the nursery. Macro scarcity influences decisions on which babies to admit to a facility. Micro scarcity is a consideration in the day-to-day, moment-to-moment decisions on which babies are to be assigned certain pieces of machinery. Only very sick babies are admitted, and, since there is more need than the hospital can meet, the sicker the baby the better the chances of admission to the nursery. There are limits, however. Some babies are so sick that they cannot benefit from therapy. These babies are not admitted. Equipment is not usually scarce inside the nursery. When need does exceed supply, however, the sicker baby again prevails, though without limits this time: whoever needs something the most—a warmer, say (a device much like a space heater that keeps babies warm)—gets it. Later I find out that scarcity is not, in this case, due to economizing. The nursery is the second most expensive unit at Northeastern Hospital (exceeded only by the critical care unit—crisis medicine at the adult level).

As we walk this afternoon, I watch nurses touching, caressing, talking to babies. Dr. Richmond tells me that the nurses work four ten-hour shifts a week. "They get attached to certain babies," Richmond says. "And they complain of stress and burn-out." There is an unreal quality about some of the babies. Some are so small that they do not look like any babies I have seen. A few weigh as little as 500 grams (just over one pound). Others appear more nearly normal. One has been in the level one wing for five months. "This is baby Michael," Richmond remarks as we pause outside of his crib. "He's dying. And it is affecting everyone." One nurse is lovingly attending to an infant smaller than any doll, gently massaging the baby's back with an electrically powered brush (like a large toothbrush).

We move slowly away to other babies. Richmond tells me of the elitism of the nurses, especially in the intensive wing of the nursery. They compete with the doctors over treatment of the babies. Is this good? Yes, Richmond answers, the competition is healthy. Nurses can and do talk with families. Sometimes they say the wrong thing, Richmond admits. They paint too bleak a picture or give the wrong information. Wrong as in incorrect, or wrong as in privileged, information? Both, Richmond answers. "But it's worth it," she says, "because of the value of such communication to both nurses and families." Many of the babies are being ventilated (given breathing help with respirators) and many are attached to intravenous units (for medicine, nourishment). Some have bandages over parts of their heads. Others are unmasked. Both white and black babies are patients. One infant (I swear) looks at me right in my eyes, though most move restlessly with their eyes shut. Many seem reddish in color to me.

The visit is over too quickly for me to absorb much. Impressions remain, strong images of a place with power and intensity and, let it be noted, a surreal quality to it. Richmond and I agree to meet the following day in her office.

January 27. A meeting with Catherine Richmond and Peggy Ryan this afternoon in Richmond's office to discuss my research in the nursery. Ryan is head of the nursing staff. She is an intelligent, tough, attractive woman in her late twenties or early thirties. She tells me that she has been working at Northeastern General for five and one-half years. "How quickly time passes when you're having fun," she adds sarcastically. She asks me who will see the results of my study. I answer, only I will on a daily basis, though a typist will transcribe the taped interviews. Then I will publish a book and hope the whole world will read the finished product. Does the hospital have to be named? No, I say. I will protect the hospital by using a fictitious name. I also pledge not to talk with parents in the nursery, though I leave open the possibility of a new research arrangement to include parents if the need arises later. (It does arise, and I do interview parents later.) We are all satisfied with the arrangements. I will have complete access to the nursery, freedom to come in at any time of the day or night and to talk to any of the staff without restrictions.

As Ryan and I walk to the nurse's station for more introductions, she asks me to wait a week until she can tell all of the nurses about me at two staff meetings to be held in the next several days. I agree. She also tells me that the busiest times in the nursery are 10:00 A.M., 1:00 P.M., and 4:00 P.M. At these three times the babies are fed, cleaned, and given their medicine. The place can get hectic anytime, however, if four to five babies are suddenly admitted at once (not an uncommon occurrence, I discover later). Both Peggy Ryan and Catherine Richmond seem to me to be thinking and working at high levels. I like them both enormously. The atmosphere here is good. My adrenalin is up for the work of the next several months.

February 7. I almost lost access to the nursery today. I went in yesterday afternoon for a 1½-hour session equipped with micro-recorder and asked many of the nurses ice-breaking questions, cute little inquiries. Several physicians stared at me. One asked me who I was. Bad vibes all around. I am in the nursery again this morning for 2½ hours. After the visit I am accosted in the hall afterwards by a formidable Dr. Margaret Grant, who tells me that she does not know who I am or what I am doing but I cannot go into the nursery with a tape recorder. She is fierce. I sweet-talk her into the conference room, where I explain my research project. She seems mollified. Later, though, Richmond calls me and tells me I am out until further notice. She suggests that I make a presentation of the research project to a meeting of the medical staff tomorrow. It seems no one told the physicians of my project. I agree to the presentation, feeling that the first pivotal situation is coming up.

Observations up to now: (1) The nurses are very affectionate with the babies. Some admit to bonding with selected infants. (2) I am not getting through in those casual interviews. So far only the cosmetic side is being presented. I have to set up other arrangements.

February 9. The presentation yesterday went well. A colleague at the university advised me to grovel before the doctors. "They like that," he said. I rejected this, not for macho reasons but because I sense my only chance is to impress as a peer. I am right, for once. They seem intrigued by the project. One doctor, however, shouts at me about confidentiality and families. "What am I to tell the parents of my patients when they ask who you are?" I stay cool, remembering old literary lore about grace under pressure. Why not—I suggest—tell them that I am a university professor doing research? Another doctor reminds the meeting of how many loose-lipped respiratory therapists parade through the nursery. Everyone seems satisfied when I agree to keep the recorder out of the nursery. (An innocuous concession, by the way. I decided two days ago to abandon the recorder on methodological grounds—it is too intrusive an instrument for use in the nursery.) I go away from the meeting optimistic about being readmitted.

Some conjectures. Most of the philosophical and legal literature tries to define a human being (or human person) in terms of criteria that entities either approximate or realize. Thus a human being is any creature who, for example, is sentient at a certain high level, or is rational in special ways, or has a certain chromosomal endowment, and so on. Something else is going on in the nursery. All of the babies in here are regarded as human beings regardless of their physical condition. Each baby is the recipient of respect, affection, and even love, from at least one nurse (and some babies—who are particularly endearing in some way—are loved by everyone). This human regard begins as soon as a baby enters the nursery. Perhaps the state of being human is a matter of location, of crossing certain physical thresholds beyond which all entrants are regarded as members of the human community because they have passed some gateway test. Or *where* a baby is located may be more decisive in her being treated as a person than *what* she is. And the same baby may not be a person outside of the nursery before admission, and may become a person by virtue of entering the nursery.

February 20. On returning from a trip to London (unrelated to the research project) I find in my mail a letter from the president of Northeastern General Hospital officially sanctioning me as an investigator in the neonatal nursery. Cheers, post facto.

February 23. I resume observations. As I enter the nursery this morning (without tape recorder) I encounter Dr. Paul Montgomery, the one who was so aggressive during the staff meeting. I open my hands to show that I have no recorder. He is especially cordial in return (to my relief), coming over to tell me in private tones how the nursery really works. Admission to the nursery is precipitated almost always by a call from an attending pediatrician. A resident neonatologist discusses the case with the pediatrician. Decision on admission is made on the inferred viability of the baby (weight plus gestational age combined with a number of clinical signs like heart and respiration rates) and, in marginal cases, the attitude of the immediate family. Montgomery tells me of a baby born last Thursday in Northeastern General to retarded parents. The baby had severe hydrocephalus (swelling in the head), a cleft palate, and no eyes (which had strong emotional effects on the staff). Montgomery talked at some level with the parents and told them that no resuscitation would be attempted unless they, the parents, wanted it. Only ordinary treatment would be pursued. After the parents had discussed the matter between themselves for two hours, they agreed with the doctors. The baby died a short time later. Montgomery on scarcity: Obstetricians want to increase the number of beds for women who may have problems in delivering their babies. The turn-around time for obstetrics beds is measured in days and weeks. But babies admitted to the nursery will tie up beds for an average of two months. Here are the seeds of a problem. Scarcity in the nursery leads Montgomery to oppose enlarging the obstetrics ward. Such are the systemic dependencies of a modern hospital.

Baby Michael lies inert as I pass his bed. He is by far the largest baby in the nursery. The staff is trying to decide whether to permit surgeons to repair his hernia.

February 24. Doctors and nurses are crowded around one of the beds. A baby has dislodged the tracheal tube that supplies him with life-retaining oxygen. "It just came off—we don't know how." The baby is being given oxygen by a mechanical respirator while one of the doctors tries to reinsert the tube. The atmosphere is light although the situation is life-threatening. "Did anyone ask him if he could breathe?" "No, but I asked him if his tube was dislodged." "And he said—I'm not the doctor, you tell me," etc. Obviously the staff is doing what all competent figures do in a tense situation, from athletes to actors to doctors—they are kidding around to stay relaxed and reduce tension. They all look pretty good as they work.

2

The demarcation between admission decisions and decisions on allocating scarce resources within the nursery is sharper now after two interviews (taped, outside the nursery but in the hospital)—one with Catherine Richmond, the other with Peggy Ryan. Admission decisions are governed by triage, a principle that selects those babies who will benefit most from treatment. Allocation decisions in the nursery are made on the basis of who needs the therapy the most, so that the sickest babies get precedence. The issue of survival does not occur in the nursery the way it does in that set of babies over which admissions decisions are made. Those outside will (usually) not survive if denied admission; and, indeed, a negative decision is strongly influenced by whether the baby has a realistic chance at survival even with aggressive therapy. Allocation decisions in the nursery are less dramatic, usually involving only delays, not life and death.

From an interview with Peggy Ryan
Frohock: Well, do you sometimes not admit babies because they may not be viable? For example, those under 500 grams?
Ryan: It has been done both ways. There are times when the doctors will say—there's nothing more we would do here.

Why go to the expense, trouble, and time, and have the end results turn out the same. Then there are the times when the physician who wants to transport the baby does not feel comfortable just sitting back doing nothing. He feels he has to do something. Depending on the doctors on service here, they may say, yes, transport the child, just to comfort the outlying hospital doctor.

Frohock: What goes into a definition of viability? Is it just weight, is it gestational age, severity of the problem, or some combination of these?

Ryan: I think it's based on the personal, ethical code of the doctor on service in combination with weight plus gestational age. What's the child clinically doing now? Does this child have a chance? There are certain—I'm trying to think of the proper word to use—there are just certain signs that point toward a good prognosis. Each time, I think, it's the weight. I remember one point years back, anything under 800 grams was not viable. Well, we've had a couple of 600-grammers who've made it. So now it's down to 500 grams. Of course, every year with modern technology, I think it's getting lower and lower.

Frohock: You said something that piqued my interest—the ethical code of the physician. What do you mean by that?

Ryan: Every person has a different theory, personally, inside their heads, as to what is viability. It's just like people saying that the quality of life is different. There are some people who do not feel as though a deformed baby should live. Then there are other people who feel as though *everything* should be done—it's still a life, and the quality of life can be improved and you don't know what the outcome is going to be. I don't think the variance among the different doctors here is as large a difference as you'll find in the spectrum of people outside. I'm sure if you asked people out there you'd get a much broader range of what people would say—"Yes, save the child," or "No, don't save the child." It's much tighter here. You understand what I'm saying?

Frohock: I understand that. I want to explore that range with you.

Ryan: But there is still a range. Small as it may be, there is still a range. Obviously, here there are four different people [neonatologists]. You're going to have four different feelings on what is viability. Is the quality of life going to play a part in what I decide to do? I'm sure they ask themselves that.

Triage can be stated simply enough: assign medical therapy to those who can best benefit from the therapy or, in more dramatic terms, to those who have the best chance for survival. Suppose that three babies need to be admitted to the nursery and, for whatever reasons, only one can be admitted. Suppose further that one is suffering from trisomy 13 (a genetic defect that is almost always fatal within a short time), the second is a victim of necrotizing enterocolitis (a disease that destroys the intestines and, if severe enough, allows children to live only for a few years), and the third is a baby born prematurely but with no significant defects other than those associated with prematurity. Triage says admit the third baby on the grounds that efforts directed at this infant are more likely to be successful.

Triage is often contrasted with a variety of moral principles urging us to help those who are worst off. Shift the terms of the example (which will almost always allow a different conclusion to be drawn). Imagine now a more demanding situation: three individuals are bleeding profusely from severe wounds incurred in an accident. One is a small child, the second an anemic adult, the third a healthy teenager. Though any number of details can change even these conclusions, triage in this case would urge concentrating attention on the healthy teenager, again because this individual has the best chance of survival. Some moral principles, however, would require assisting the adult on the grounds that he is the worst off of the three. The moral imperative becomes stronger if the physical condition is caused by unjust treatment. Imagine, for example, that the adult's anemia developed while he was incarcerated unjustly for a long period.

Other principles of choice can conflict with both triage and morality. Social utility, both host and antagonist of moral choice, can bid us to select the individual who can contribute most to society. On a simple calculation of probable life spans, we might still choose to help the teenager on the grounds that he is at the threshold of an independent and, one would hope, productive life. Here is where the power of examples to control argument can be seen. If the small child (in a redescription of the situation) is a mathematics prodigy, then efforts to maximize utility might compel saving this individual rather than the other two.

Triage provides a logic of choice for limited resources. It fails badly in conditions of abundance, especially when the items to be allocated are life-maintaining goods. Again change the example.

Now suppose that the three individuals are all patients in a modern hospital and ill with bacterial infections. Should penicillin be given only, or even first, to the one who is healthiest on the grounds that such an individual is more likely to be cured by the therapy? No one in medicine today would subscribe to such a policy. The appropriate ranking of the individuals is by need.

Triage is the guiding principle for admission to the nursery. Need dominates allocation decisions within the nursery. Why? The most obvious explanation is scarcity. Not every baby can be admitted to the nursery. But once in, there are enough items to meet the most pressing needs in therapy. There is a more intriguing explanation, however. Perhaps babies not yet admitted do not constitute a human community in the eyes of physicians, while those within the nursery do. This explanation would explain admission denials when scarcity is not crucial, since triage used toward nonhuman forms of life does not seem so morally controversial. No gateway decision is more profound, if true; for the admission decision is then a decision on who is to count as human.

There is more of interest here. Ryan says that the moral principles held by physicians influence judgments on viability. Are determinations of physical conditions controlled by the physician's subscription to some vision of a good or worthwhile life?

3

March 1. I had an interview yesterday with Bill Camisa, one of the two residents. He tells me they can bring a peach back from the dead with the skills they have developed. I also spent some time observing in the nursery. Two items: (1) I am becoming more convinced that there is no absolute or overarching definition of a human being in use here—that definitions vary within sectors of medical practices. (2) People are so emotional about these issues that moral posturing rather than rational discourse is the norm. The latter item is drawn from my experience at a campus seminar on euthanasia. One of the participants kept drawing parallels between the Holocaust and current practices in neonatal units. I responded with the obligatory rudeness that seems to characterize sessions like these. People simply are not thinking on these problems. The question is, am I?

A nurse tells me today that if she had her way, no twenty-four-week (gestation-age) babies would be admitted to the nursery. She says that they are too premature to make it. Earlier than that point they do not even have lungs.

Again I see a baby stop breathing. The alarm on the respirator machine (a gentle sound, much like a snooze reminder) goes off, and the nurse, after shutting off the alarm, prods the baby back to life by pushing and rubbing his tiny body. During this resuscitation she talks to him with rough affection: "Come on, dummy. Why did you do that? Quit it. Don't you know any better than to stop breathing?" I ask why he stopped breathing. She answers, "Prematurity." And tells me that this problem will go away once he matures a bit.

How can I introduce these experiences to the philosophical literature on human identity?

March 2. I continue to tape interviews with individual members of the staff. They are beginning to speak to me about their personal feelings on euthanasia and quality-of-life considerations in therapy.

Nothing exceptional is happening today in the nursery. Susan Markart, one of the neonatologists, tells me it is unusually calm, not at all a real picture of how things are most of the time. Bill Camisa invites me to make morning rounds with him tomorrow.

March 5. I am in the hospital this morning at 7:20 A.M. for morning rounds at 7:30 A.M. But there are no morning rounds today because the staff are occupied with more pressing matters. A three-day-old baby has a pneumothorax, which is a sudden release of air from the lungs to an area outside of the lungs. It is dangerous and will kill the child quickly unless treated. Camisa and other doctors stabilize the infant in a standard way, by withdrawing the excessive air in the sack outside of the lungs and inserting a new (and this time larger) breathing tube. There is also talk of the imminent arrival of premature twins (boys) who are being delivered by cesarian section at twenty-eight weeks' gestation. I am so fascinated by all the activity that I call over to the university and cancel my office hours for this morning. I must stay and see what is going on.

I talk with Rebecca Smith, a nurse who has been in the hospital for eight years except for one ten-month stint elsewhere and one leave of absence to have a baby of her own. She says that the nurses do almost everything in the level 2 unit (the less-intensive area) because the doctors are not interested in nonacute babies. "They just don't bother to go in there very much." Her "baby"—the one she is caring for—has just been moved across the hall to make room for one of the twins. Her own child is in a day-care center while she and her husband work. The phone rings while we talk. Smith shouts "Mash unit. Incoming wounded." And sure enough the call is an announcement that the twenty-eight week twins are on the way up.

This place is a magnet to me. I can't pull myself away. Why? Because it is like going in the best magic room at the state fair with all the latest lights and equipment and magicians performing fantastic tricks with the highest-priced prizes at stake—health, life. And because, unlike most high-technology centers (which are cold places), this place is filled with human love. Babies, all babies, can do this to a place—and they are doing it here (their own magic).

I am in the hospital briefly this afternoon. All the doctors and interns are in the daily X-ray session (reviewing films on the babies). There is also a power outage. Only a reserve generator is supplying electricity. This means, among other things, that the nurses have to ventilate the babies manually. Many lights are cut off to save power. Some parents are present, looking more than normally worried. I decide to return to my office, leaving a message to Drs. Markart and Schwartz to call me if they are free for interviews. As I leave, fire engines pull up with sirens roaring, lights flashing. I ask a police officer outside the hospital what the problem is. He waves me off with his hand. After he turns around I send my own hand signal back to him. Then I follow the firemen in and ask another policeman what is going on. He tells me that the heat indicators in the basement triggered the fire alarm, probably because the power outage has cut off the air conditioning. I walk back to the campus, musing (as we all must) on the compensatory functions of modern technology.

These preliminaries from the study so far: Ordinary care for the baby means receiving (1) fluids, (2) warmth, and (3) food. Extraordinary care is anything beyond these three items. This interesting caveat, however: warmth hastens death in a dying infant. So comfort, in extreme cases, is a slide toward the grave.

Like most professionals, doctors deem the brain the most important organ to have intact. Life is worth living if there is at least enough of a functioning brain to relate to other people, and perhaps also some bodily mobility (so that the patient is not tied to beds,

support systems, etc.). Would beauty contest winners rank morphology above neurology? Parents, I am told, invariably ask about
the neurological functions of their stricken children before anything
else.

> *From an interview with Dr. Susan Markart. Markart is in her
> mid-thirties. She has been a neonatologist in the nursery for only five
> years, but her reputation with the staff is exceedingly high. Included
> among her considerable skills is a legendary ability to find—al-
> ways—a vein in any child for a needle or I.V.*

Frohock: Do you have any thoughts about what makes a life worth
living that you might consider in making hard choices about
therapy?

Markart: I guess it's a long discussion actually.

Frohock: We have time. I do.

Markart: I guess there has to be some ability to react to your environment. It may sound silly or simplistic, but the ability
to smile. For a child to be able to smile at his parents is
absolutely important to his ability to interact. Having a baby
that is never even going to be able to smile because his brain
doesn't communicate that well with the environment—I
think that's a child who is not perhaps viable or worth saving
in the long term. A child who is tied to a ventilator, who is
tied to machinery for the rest of his life, or has to spend his life
in an institution because he can never be cared for at home—
that's a great flaw in his life. The child who even is just tied to
a bed and has such severe mental retardation that he can't
handle his own secretions. One who has to be fed, his body
all twisted up, depending on everyone else without any
interaction with his parents. If I knew that was going to be the
future, that is a child I would not be aggressive with.

A baby was born a few months ago in the hospital who had no
brain. He had a brain stem which controlled respiration and heart
rates. So the possibility existed for a "viable" child without a brain
living for months, perhaps years, as a vegetable. The physicians
attached an I.V. but then, in consultation with the parents, decided
not to connect the baby to a ventilator. The child died in two days.

Dr. Joseph Schwartz, an intern who is completing his duties in
the nursery in a few weeks, tells me that he wanted to avoid even
placing the I.V. in the child, which made the other doctors look at
him strangely. They viewed the denial of an I.V. as active euthana-

sia. Schwartz's point is that it was only a step down, one notch less in the scale of aggressive therapy. I ask the obvious question—Why not give the child an injection immediately for a quick, painless death? Schwartz answers that he would favor it, but would never consider doing such a thing in the current legal and moral climate in the country. Then Schwartz mentions *Of Mice and Men* to me. He asks me if killing Lennie was wrong. If not, then surely it is right to pull the plug in extreme cases.

Here is the conundrum Schwartz communicates to me. Suppose that 95 percent of babies who are under twenty-five weeks' gestation will develop into comatose adults whose lives are without any human qualities at all, but that 5 percent of under-twenty-five-week babies will lead reasonably good lives. Now let's say we cannot tell which of the babies will be in the 5 percent to pass beyond some quality threshold for human life. A refusal to treat all under-twenty-five-week infants will result in the deaths of the 5 percent along with the 95 percent. But if it is impossible to terminate aggressive therapy once it has begun, then we face the spectacle of 95 percent of this class of babies living on life-support systems for years as severely brain-damaged individuals, unaware of their environment and in constant discomfort and even pain. It follows that there is a rational incentive in medicine to deny treatment to all under-twenty-five-week babies. Query: which is better: no treatment at all for under-twenty-five-week babies, or treatment of all under-twenty-five-week babies with passive or active euthanasia later of the 95 percent who fall below some critical quality threshold?

Frohock: Suppose you are faced with a hard decision like that on whether to continue aggressive therapy. Would the legal implications, the possibility of charges being brought, be the primary consideration in your thinking?

Schwartz: Well, you see it's not that hard a decision anymore because there's really no decision. The people just are not doing it. What they're doing is, in my opinion, even worse. What they're doing right now is trying to figure out when do we begin to act aggressively. Let's say someone is a drowning victim. Right now we are trying to develop criteria—when do you start aggressive resuscitation? If they have been under water for x amount of minutes, statistically it shows that they are going to end up with a lot of neurologic sequelae, so we are not even going to bother with aggressive treatment. But that's silly. What we should be doing is giving everyone a chance in my opinion. If it doesn't pan out, then pull the plug. Then stop the respiratory support. But now what we do is either we don't start because we think in the majority it is going to be a poor prognosis, and if we do start, if they end up in a very bad shape neurologically and on a respirator assumingly for life, we just leave them there. To me it's aesthetically and ethically really distasteful to leave people in this sort of situation. If it was my kid, if it was myself, I would certainly wish myself and my child dead. But we are not allowed to pull the plug and it's not left up to the physician or the family.

Schwartz also tells me that he is so disgusted with pediatric medicine at this level that he is changing his specialty to dermatology.

Reflections at the end of a day: Am I seeing everything? So far I have not seen any baby die or any extreme cases. Am I being kept away from certain critical areas of medical practice in the nursery?

2
Hard Cases

1

One of the striking visual features of the nursery is the organized cheerfulness of the decor. The main hall is kept freshly painted in white, with multicolored balloons painted on the walls on both sides. On the wall in one of the rooms is a large lion decal. The lion has pink skin and a yellow mane. On the opposite wall is a stuffed clown with three balloons. Underneath the clown is a message from a former patient: "Thank you, love always, Susan Bendix." In another room there is a wall decal of a yellow elephant with pink ears, and on a side wall hangs an actual striped kite with bows on the tail. One of the beds in this room contains a stuffed bear. A nurse turns over the baby on the bed and winds up the bear, which emits soft music.

March 8. I was in the unit this morning for almost three hours and saw a dreadful yet fascinating case. A baby, Stephanie Christopher, was born at 2:00 A.M. today in the hospital. She is premature (thirty weeks in term). But her main problem is that she is afflicted with a congenital disorder, epidermolysis bullosa, that causes widespread and constant blistering of the skin. There is no scarring in the version that Stephanie has, but the lesions occur both on the outer surface of the body and on skin within the body, such as the mouth and esophagus. Secondary growth retardation and severe anemia are part of the syndrome. The pathogenesis is unknown. The disease is caused by a recessive gene in both parents, which, when present, leads to the malady in one-fourth of the parents' offspring. The "prognosis is grave," according to Abraham M. Rudolph's *Pediatrics* (17th edition), and "many succumb to the disease or its complications within the first two years." The doctors attending baby Stephanie tell me that they have seen only one child with the disease (a less severe form than Stephanie has) live to adulthood.

Stephanie is in reverse isolation (since the major cause of death in these children is infection). Nurses caring for her must wear sterile gowns, masks, and caps to avoid contaminating her environment. In the nursery I don the required outfit and enter her room. I am told that all of Stephanie's cognitive faculties are present. She is very alert, though how much of this is due to the stimulation of pain I do not know. She keeps jerking her limbs restlessly every few minutes. Whenever the nurse touches her she cries. Efforts to clear her tracheal and bronchial tubes with suction and sterile water bring up traces of blood. Treatment at the moment consists of antibiotics and fluids (via an I.V.). No respirator is in evidence and there is no breathing distress. Stephanie's skin has many blisters. She is a lovely girl, with delicate features. I am told that she is the third child of the parents. The first had the same disorder and lived six weeks. The second is free of the disease. The mother went to a university hospital in her sixth month of pregnancy for a biopsy of the fetus. Something went wrong with the test and the results were inconclusive. She decided to continue the pregnancy. The baby also has an intestinal obstruction that prevents feeding (a problem often associated with the disease). The obstruction must be corrected surgically if the child is to live any length of time at all.

The nurse caring for Stephanie is terribly moved by the baby. She tells me that it's hard, that it tears her to pieces. "I wouldn't have children if I had this gene." Even at 1–4 odds? "No. I've seen too many of these children. I wouldn't do it to my child."

I leave Stephanie's room and, in the hall, see the dermatologist who has been called in as a consultant on the case. "I know what I would have done," he says. "I wouldn't have treated her." Who should make this decision? "Good question. Parents, probably." Then, in a spontaneous moment of candor, he tells me that one of his own children was born with a severe genetic disorder. He decided not to treat. The baby died quickly. I ask him what he considered in making the decision. He lists these: future pain ("The current pain is not important; there is no memory of pain at this age"), what the disease would have done to other children in his family (he had three other children at the time), and the type of life (he judged it not worth living).

Questions to myself: If there is no memory of pain, does pain not exist at the time it is supposedly occurring? Does human experience require memory to be human experience? If this is so, then what is baby Stephanie experiencing when she writhes "in pain." Or is such a young baby not human? Not a person? Is this implied by the dermatologist's observation on pain?

March 9. Susan Markart tells me as I walk in that "we have the biggest moral problem of the century." It seems that she has done some research on Stephanie's disease and found a therapeutic treatment requiring a Clinitron bed that allows the baby to float on a type of air mattress. The bed is also a heating unit. Numerous small spheres of silicone are kept aloft and warm by a continual flow of hot air. A sheet is placed on the spheres and the baby rests on the floating cloth. There are only two such beds for babies in the country. The manufacturers are willing to fly one of the beds to Northeastern without charge. But Nursing Services (a part of the hospital's administration) has balked at the daily costs. The bed rents for $65 a day, an expense not covered by Medicaid. Markart is angry. She asks the administrator who has rejected the request for the bed if she wants to write that medical judgment on the patient's chart or would she prefer to tell Stephanie's mother herself. Everyone keeps telling me that $65 a day is two blood gases. In other words, peanuts. Interesting. What if the cost were $6,500 a day? Or $65,000?

A nurse tells me the story of a hospital administrator who would not permit the letters "E.T." (which the nurses were using as an abbreviation for endocarditis—an inflammation of the cardiac connective tissue) on beds because she thought the babies did look like the extra terrestrial character E.T. The nurse uses the story to illustrate the insanity of administrators.

A "Do we have a porta-potty" sign is on the window of the isolation room containing Stephanie. The nurse inside, Rebecca Smith, says through her sterile mask: "I'm hot, I'm tired." Later, at lunch, I ask her what bothers her the most about treating babies like Stephanie. She answers: "First, it messes up your hair. I had a perm this morning and now look at my hair. Trivial, but it's something. Second, you can't do the procedures as well with the gloves on. You always worry, I'm going to break the sterilization and kill the child with an infection. Third, the child itself—its suffering. I would have my tubes tied before I'd allow a child of mine to suffer like that." Even with the odds against the disease? "Yes—I'd have my tubes tied. No children." What do you do to relax? "I can't talk about my work with my husband. He doesn't understand. No one can who doesn't know the work. Sometimes I get together with the other nurses and we just talk about all the problems. Get it all out. I sew a lot. I like that. And every Thursday a bunch of us girls get together with our children and just talk and let the kids run wild. That's a good time."

March 11. Susan Markart calls me at 6:45 A.M. today (Sunday) and asks me if I want to see some interesting new arrivals. I say yes, quickly shower, and then eat breakfast with Chrissy (my younger daughter), who has also been invited. Chrissy is only twelve years old but wants to study medicine. Markart asks me to bring her along "to nurture a future pediatrician." We arrive at Northeastern General at 7:45 A.M. on a cold, blustery day.

The first case is a fetus (the staff's term here) born at twenty-five weeks, 580 grams. No spontaneous breathing occurred at birth. Only a mild heartbeat could be detected. Bruises all over the body. A swollen head (as if from intracranial bleeding). Pallid—almost gray. A very thin umbilical cord suggesting restricted nutrition throughout gestation. In general, not a promising baby. Markart decided on the spot in the delivery room not to resuscitate. She placed the baby on cloth wraps to die. It had expired by the time I reached the nursery. A nurse was crying. "The mother," she said, "had already named it." It looked to me like a miniature replica of a baby asleep (hands folded under its face, lying on its side) though without any color or, of course, life. Did this baby live? Does such a question make sense? The mother refused the postmortem that Markart suggested as a basis for future genetic counseling. Afterwards, one of the fourth-year medical students sits down with me and tells me that she was in the delivery room and everyone on the staff was relieved when Susan made the decision not to resuscitate. To me, this death—if it can be called that—was as nothing compared to the death of a whole mature person. Is human identity properly assigned to the sentient side of human life? Is a person's soul formed from experience rather than conception? The sorrow here was with the adults, the emotional pain with the family of the infant—or those with mature brains who are fully conscious of life and have lived through experiences. I steal a final glance at the little girl. She is wrapped in white cloth, the cloth pinned in the front with a large, amber-colored safety pin.

The second case is a full-term baby born with possible neurological problems. Cindy Blackwell is the baby's name. Her pupils do not constrict when light is shined on them (though apparently this lack of response in a baby does not mean what it decidedly does mean in an adult: brain death). She also has apnea (she stops breathing) when she falls asleep. The CAT scan shows no significant abnormalities in the brain, though it picks up some peculiarities (such as an extraordinarily thick skull). The father of the child has a family history of neurological problems. Markart is waiting for a more experienced person to read the CAT scan. Then, in twenty-four hours or so, she will call in a neurologist to examine the child.

The third case is a baby weighing only 700 grams. She is named Danielle Raymond and is from a small village about sixty miles from Northeastern. The mother had told the obstetrician at her local hospital that she was seventeen weeks pregnant, though she was actually twenty-six to twenty-seven weeks in term. At the delivery the obstetrician assumes that he is dealing with a miscarriage and leaves the baby on a table to expire. A priest comes over to baptize the baby and notices movement. Resuscitation efforts begin fourteen minutes after the birth (a lifetime—literally—for a baby in this condition). She is rushed by helicopter to Northeastern's neonatal unit, where, in the words of Susan Markart, "full-court press, all-out" efforts begin. Mucus is plugging up the baby's bronchial tubes on arrival and there is possible asphyxia and consequent brain damage. One of the Fellows in the nursery tells me he rates the baby's chances at 50–50. After cleaning her bronchial tubes and stabilizing her, the staff decides to "sit on it" for twenty-four hours. There is talk of a blood transfusion for the baby in the next hour, however. Danielle's mother does not want her. The father is indifferent.

Rebecca Smith, the nurse on duty with baby Stephanie, comes up to me. "Do you know what she tried to pull just now? She kicked out her I.V. and lost one-third of her blood before we could get another one in." The problem is that the I.V. cannot penetrate more than a short distance. Also it must be inserted in her abdomen because of the skin lesions. The doctors and nurses have restabilized her by 8:00 A.M. Smith: "I need a whiskey." I ask her if that is the drug of choice for the nurses. "It is for me."

The doctors and nurses are talking to me now, and even seeking me out to show me things. I am grateful of course. But why are they doing it? My conjectures: (1) to show off their professional skills; (2) to make a case for their own interests against others, especially the state—the doctors think they are right in what they do and want someone to represent their views in public, to state their side of things; and (3) to ask for help, for while carrying a torch of righteousness they are also genuinely concerned about some of the complex ethical issues they are encountering.

Susan Markart, Chrissy, and I visit the eighth floor of Northeastern, where the obstetrics wing is located. Normal and healthy babies are everywhere. The differences couldn't be greater. The only sounds are the lusty cries of babies. No machines are in evidence. There is also a quiet, relaxed atmosphere—no one seems in a rush to do anything. No emergencies, in short. Now I see the only mechanical device around—a scale to weigh the babies. Health, I think, is like a mirror, always deflecting attention from itself to other things. Illness, in contrast, is a vortex of activity that seems to demand increasingly intense attention for its own sake. Also, the healthy babies up here on these floors will look at you, make eye contact. Not the ones below in the nursery.

March 12. Stephanie throws off her I.V. again this morning. Again it is reattached by the doctors. She also suffers from asphyxia, caused by the clogging of her trachea. The nurse swears she turns black every thirty minutes and must be suctioned clear like clockwork on the half hour. The epidermis separates from the dermis in this condition, so Stephanie's skin is constantly sloughing off throughout the respiratory tract and digestive system. Surgery is still being contemplated to correct the intestinal obstruction, though there will be difficult postoperative healing problems. Stephanie needs a tube now to help her breathe, but the doctors cannot insert it because her internal skin will slough off when the device touches it. One piece of good news: Nursing Services has relented and the special bed is on the way.

Later in the day Stephanie has brief bouts of apnea. She is given oxygen via a mask near her face. She is also losing weight, from 1240 grams at birth to today's 1220 grams. Her treatment still consists of short courses of antibiotics. Frequent cultures are drawn to see what organisms may be present in her body. Vaseline gauzes are being applied to the blisters on her skin. Some of the doctors discuss the legal issues if the parents refuse surgery for her. A nurse says a refusal is possible "if everyone keeps quiet about it." The recent Baby Doe case is discussed.

2

The Baby Doe case mentioned by the staff at Northeastern began in the fall of 1983. (For literature on the case, see the Bibliography, section 2.) An infant was born on October 11 in Port Jefferson, Long Island, suffering from spina bifida, hydrocephalus, and microcephalus. Spina bifida is a condition in which the spinal cord fails to close properly; hydrocephalus is an excess of fluid in the brain; microcephalus is a small head. The seriousness of spina bifida depends on where the opening to the spinal cord occurs; higher openings are proportionately more serious. The medical treatment most commonly pursued is to close the opening surgically, though the prognosis after surgery varies considerably. Some spina bifida patients lead nearly normal lives after surgery. Others are severely retarded and immobile for the remainder of their lives. Some die in spite of surgical efforts. Where the opening occurs—whether high or low—is again important in determining the short- and long-range prognosis for a baby. It is important to note that from the beginning of the Baby Doe case to its final resolution the location of the baby's spinal opening was never made public.

Doctors who examined the baby, identified only as Baby Jane Doe, said that without surgery the infant would die in two years. With surgery she could survive into her twenties but would be severely retarded and bedridden. The parents of the baby, after consulting with neurologists, social workers, clergymen, and family, decided against surgery to close the spinal opening and, in a second operation, to drain fluid from the brain. They claimed that the attending physician had told them that the two operations carried risks to the baby, including paralysis and the loss of bladder and rectal functions. The doctors and the hospital administrators abided by the parents' wishes. No surgery was contemplated and the hospital continued conservative medical care of the child (which included the use of antibiotics).

Four days after the parents' decision, however, a right-to-life attorney, acting on a tip from someone on the hospital staff, intervened. Lawrence Washburn, a private attorney in Albany with offices in New York City, sued the hospital to force corrective surgery for the opening to the spine. The case was unprecedented in several respects. Washburn had never met the parents nor seen either the baby or the baby's hospital records. He was in all respects an outsider with no direct interests in the case. Nevertheless he argued that the baby's life was at stake if he did not act immediately.

The basis of the suit was also unusual. Washburn claimed that the case was one of discrimination—that the baby was being denied surgery because she was born handicapped. The handicaps in this case were spina bifida, hydrocephalus, and microcephalus. In subsequent weeks Washburn expanded his suit to include the parents, the New York attorney general, and the State Department of Social Services.

The New York Court of Appeals, on October 28, 1983, upheld the parents' right to forgo surgery for their daughter. The court, in a unanimous opinion, affirmed this right with strong language, describing the lawsuit challenging the right as "unusual" and "offensive" and stating that "the hearing court abused its discretion" in permitting the case to go forward. The appeals court stated that the petitioner (Washburn) "had no direct interest in or relationship to any party" (the child, parents, family, physicians) and that it found it "distressing" that the parents, in addition to their anguish over the birth of a child with severe physical disorders, also were subject to weeks of litigation "through all three levels of our state's court system." The appeals court did, however, treat the case as a procedural matter, holding that the proper course of action for such cases was not through the legal system but through child protection agencies under appropriate provisions of the Family Court Act.

A few days later the federal government filed suit to force the hospital to turn over the medical records on Baby Jane Doe. A White House aide was quoted as saying that presidential counselor Edwin Meese personally approved the federal government's intervention in the case. The government said that it wanted to determine whether the baby was a victim of discrimination because she was handicapped. The Justice Department contended that the hospital, in receiving Medicaid and Medicare money, was obligated to allow government officials to inspect its records even over the objections of parents. The stick wielded by the government in its arguments was substantial. The hospital was facing the prospect of losing $20–25 million a year if it refused a court order to reveal the records.

The issues separating the adversaries in this dispute were drawn from mutually opposed principles. The government maintained that the rights of individuals to medical care, and even to life itself, override the discretionary authority of parents over the welfare of their children. Dr. C. Everett Koop, the U.S. surgeon general, said that "if we do not intrude into the life of a child such as this, whose civil rights may be abrogated, the next person may be you. We're not just fighting for this baby. We're fighting for a principle of this country that every life is individually and uniquely sacred" (*New York Times*, November 7, 1983). Precedents exist for overriding parental authority in medical therapy. Physicians can and do initiate legal proceedings to mandate medical treatment for children against their parents' wishes. In a typical case, doctors at the State University at Stony Brook, New York, obtained a court order in early 1984 authorizing a blood transfusion during surgery for the four-month-old son of a Jehovah's Witness. The mother objected to the surgery because it would require transfusions, and transfusions were forbidden by her religion. The surgery was needed to preserve the infant's life. The state supreme court overrode the mother's objections. What made the government's actions unusual in the Baby Jane Doe case was that most previous efforts to oppose the wishes of parents had been initiated by physicians on medical grounds. The government was acting in this case against a decision made by parents as well as physicians in agreement with each other.

Opponents to the government's intervention stressed the privacy of medical practice and the needs of parents to be shielded from government regulation in deciding on medical care for their children. The state attorney general's office called the government's action an extraordinary intrusion into the physician-patient privilege. Richard Rifton of the New York attorney general's office, representing the hospital in the case, argued that the government had no right to "meddle" in the case. "There is a question of fairness," he said (*New York Times*, November 5, 1983). "This issue is one of great importance to the state hospital, to hospitals throughout the country, to the medical profession and to the public at large—for any of us may be the next parents of a Baby Jane Doe." The father of the baby said that "for someone to walk in and invite the rest of the country into our house is a terrible intrusion into our lives."

On November 17, 1983, a federal district court denied the government's request to review the medical records of Baby Jane Doe. Judge Leonard Wexler rejected the government's contention that the hospital had discriminated against the baby. He said that records from the state lawsuit showed that the decision of the parents and the hospital was a reasonable one "based on due consideration of the medical options available and on a genuine concern for the best interests of the child." The Justice Department, which had never before sued to obtain access to a hospital's medical records, appealed the decision. William Bradford Reynolds, head of the department's civil rights division, said that "the shield of parental non-consent is not so impenetrable that it can foreclose all inquiry into the hospital's role regarding the treatment or lack thereof of an infant patient submitted to its care" (*Syracuse Post Standard*, November 22, 1983).

The Washburn lawsuit, in the meantime, reached the U.S. Supreme Court on appeal. There it received a short and negative response. The justices, without comment, let stand the New York court's ruling upholding the right of the parents to decide on therapy for their daughter. Washburn was not through, however. Two days before Christmas he filed a new, class action lawsuit seeking again to have the child's medical records opened and asking that a guardian be appointed for the child. A federal judge denied Washburn's suit and fined the lawyer $500 under an infrequently used federal rule permitting fines on lawyers trying to "harass or cause unnecessary delay or needlessly increase the costs of litigation." Shortly after the ruling on Washburn's latest suit, a United States appeals panel in Manhattan upheld the lower court ruling barring the federal government from examining Baby Jane Doe's medical records. The appeals court held, in a 2–1 vote, that the law against discrimination invoked by the government was never intended by Congress to "apply to treatment decisions involving defective newborn infants."

In spite of the consistent rulings by various courts against the government, however, the Justice Department went forward. It asked the appeals court to reconsider its decision. At the moment when doctors at Northeastern hospital are trying to decide on treatment for baby Stephanie, the federal government is still trying to get at the records of Baby Jane Doe, and the parents and hospital are still resisting these efforts.

3

The government and the parents in the Baby Jane Doe case are each drawing on different philosophies of decision making. The government's claim (and, to some degree, the right-to-life attorney's) is informed by the impartial-spectator model of decisions. Long traditions of social thought support this model, from Hume (especially) to the present time. The guiding thought here is that decisions on medical therapy can be more rational if supervised, and perhaps even made, by those who are not vitally linked to the child. The parents of Baby Jane Doe are relying on an affected-interest model of decision making. Here the thought is that those most strongly affected by a decision, with special interests in the outcome, ought to have their opinions weigh more heavily. Affection and commitment, not distance, are said to be the best guarantees that the interests of an individual will be respected. On this model the parents, who are presumed to love the child and see its health as one of their own vital interests, are the best judges of medical treatment. Much of recent democratic practice, a form of government that assumes an individual knows best what his own interests are, relies on an affected-interest account of decision making.

Which philosophy is more persuasive? The accounts are mixed, in and out of balance on a number of issues. In an ideal world, parents would be the best representatives of their children's interests and would always make decisions on therapy in the best interests of the child. But we do not, as we all know, live in an ideal world. Some parents are not able or willing to see their children's best interests. Cases of child abuse and neglect are daily testimonies to parental deficiencies. Legal challenges of religious beliefs that impede treatment of children suggest that even good parents can misconstrue the interests of their children. But is a distant party like the government the alternative to parental authority? Robert A. Burt, professor of law and medicine at the Yale Law School, said in an interview during the early stages of the dispute: "I like the idea that someone is looking over the decision-making. What I don't like is the Government is always going to say treat, treat, treat. That is not always the correct ethical response in all matters" (*New York Times*, November 8, 1983).

One nagging thought about the Baby Jane Doe case is that there might not be any right answers in the dispute. No evidence was ever presented to suggest that the parents of the little girl were negligent or in any way irrational. No unusual superstitions or religious beliefs inform their views. They are Catholics who assert that religion played no part in their decision. They seem in all respects genuinely concerned with the welfare of their child. The treatment they chose was conservative, ruling out those surgical interventions which would repair the spinal opening and drain the fluid from the brain. It is true that the surgery would have prolonged the life of the child and that the parents may have decided against surgery on the expectation that the child would then die very quickly. But the parents may have been prepared to say that a short life with higher quality is better than a long life with severe disabilities. The right-to-life attorney, of course, maintained that life itself is an overriding value, no matter how it is lived. But can we say with any assurance that he is right and the parents wrong? Or that the parents are right and the attorney wrong?

If reasonable people can reach different conclusions, then procedure becomes important in making decisions. In January 1984 the Reagan administration reached a compromise over the care of handicapped infants. The administration backed away from its more demanding efforts to review immediately the records of cases where parents forgo surgery or other forms of therapy. These efforts had required hospitals to post a notice containing several "hotline" phone numbers to report suspected cases of nontreatment (a practice struck down by a U.S. district court judge in the spring of 1983). The new, more moderate, approach of the government still required hospitals to post a notice, but the notice recommends that first calls go to the hospital's "infant care review committee." Then, if necessary, the routine suggests calling the state child protection agency and, finally, the federal Department of Health and Human Services. The main compromise in this approach was the unspoken assumption that hospital infant care review committees will take on the main procedural burden of negotiating disputes over medical therapy.

It was in the context of these events, and with the notice required by the government posted on the wall opposite the nurse's station in the level 1 wing of the nursery in Northeastern General, that the staff informally discussed the medical treatment for baby Stephanie. Predicting which way the decision would go on corrective surgery for the intestinal obstruction was fairly easy. The government's efforts on the New York Baby Jane Doe case was inspired in part by an earlier Doe case. A baby born in Bloomington, Indiana, in 1982 had Down's syndrome and a defective esophagus. The parents decided against surgery to correct the esophagus. The child, who could not eat with the defective esophagus, starved to death a day after the Indiana Supreme Court upheld the parents' decision. It was this ghastly event (there are no kind words to describe it) that led the Reagan administration to require hotline phone numbers in neonatology nurseries. It was a safe bet that no child would ever die again in a hospital from an obstruction preventing nourishment.

The bet is a lock. Stephanie has additional problems. There is a sterilization failure when her central venous line (for feeding) is reinserted, and no one can get monitors on her body. Also there is continued concern over infection, though none of the cultures have grown. The antibiotics are stopped for fear of promoting the growth of resistant organisms or encouraging a fungal overgrowth. But surgery is scheduled for the day after tomorrow to correct the intestinal obstruction.

Stephanie is so interesting and attractive that one forgets that the nursery is filled with other babies. A new arrival, Miguel Santana, is a full-term baby who was fine at birth. Then he started grunting, turned pale and even blue over parts of his body. The doctors rushed him down from obstetrics to the nursery. Bill Camisa stands staring at him as the nurses hook up the monitors and begin to take blood for tests. "A big blue baby," he muses. The nurses around his bed say several times that he is near a drafty window. They always complain about this particular location in the nursery. I can't feel any draft.

Cindy Blackwell, the baby suspected of having a neurological disease, is still a mystery. The CAT scan cannot adequately pick up the back of her brain (where the brain stem is located). Susan Markart is still convinced that there is some neurological problem. But whether it is diffuse or local is not clear. A neurologist is to look at the child this afternoon.

The nursery has three methods to help babies breathe better. The most innocuous is a hood, which, when placed over the baby's head, delivers supplemental oxygen for the baby to inhale. The second step up from the hood is the CPAP, which is attached to the nose and hoses oxygen up the nostrils under pressure. The most aggressive device is the ventilator. It is a machine that actually does the breathing for the baby by delivering oxygen directly to the lungs via a tube in a rhythm set to mimic breathing. The ventilator pressure settings vary from 1 to 100. Baby Danielle is on a ventilator that is set at 5.

Michael Anthony, the older baby, is back in the regular wing after a brief stay in isolation to clear up an infection he caught (and that he might have transmitted to the other babies). I am told that all babies who stay in the nursery for any length of time get infections eventually. Michael has been in the nursery for almost six months now. He is heavy. As a normal baby he would be considered chunky, maybe too bulky. In the nursery he is a giant. His face has jowls, his eyelids are thick. He has a long suture up the middle of his abdomen from earlier surgery. He is still on a ventilator. No surgery is planned at the moment, not even the hernia operation contemplated earlier.

The attire in the nursery varies. The interns wear blue-green V-neck shirts (short-sleeved) and elastic trousers (both sexes). The nurses wear white dresses. The doctors wear white smocks over their street clothes. From time to time, doctors from a private practice breeze in for a visit. They are brisk and wear shirts as white as phosphorus. Their shoes are always shined. They look like, and probably are, especially successful businessmen.

An I.V. is started in the Santana baby to give him antibiotics. Bill Camisa has trouble inserting the needle. He keeps sticking the baby's arm without finding a vein. "Unbelievable that this baby is so deep." An intern scoffs, "I've heard that line before." The intern then tries and fails. A nurse gets the I.V. in on the first try. The group of doctors walks off, already absorbed with other matters. The nurse calls out sarcastically, "I'll get the mess."

The X-rays of the Santana baby arrive. They are so bad technically that no evaluation can be made.

One of the interns has a hoarse cough. She finally puts on a surgical mask at 10:00 A.M.

I go to lunch at the hospital cafeteria with several nurses. They tell me it is impossible for anyone who is a strict right-to-lifer to work in the nursery. If you are one, you will change your views after being there a short while. All the nurses talking to me believe that the quality of life is important in deciding whether a life is worth living and a baby worth saving.

An incident occurred a few years ago at Northeastern General that is still discussed by the staff. A baby born prematurely in an outside hospital had birth asphyxia. During transport to Northeastern General the child had two cardiac arrests with major efforts made at resuscitation. In the neonatal nursery the child was put on very high ventilator support. He developed hyaline membrane disease (a disease of the lungs that inhibits growth and even breathing) and, later, interstitial emphysema (an overexpansion of the lungs where air invades space between normal lung matter rather than staying in the air sacs). One treatment for interstitial emphysema is to lower the air pressure in the lungs as aggressively as possible (which will momentarily maintain blood oxygen and blood carbon dioxide levels). On one particular day in the life of this child, after he had been in the nursery for three weeks, Kent Philips, the attending physician, tried this treatment. The baby's pH at that time was 7.1, the PCO_2 was bordering on 100, and the PO_2 was down in the 30s at 100 percent oxygen. Philips and the other doctors decided that the only chance the child had was to lower the air pressure, and so Philips reduced the ventilator setting.

Unfortunately, the nurse caring for the child (who had gotten quite attached to him) was at lunch when Philips acted. When she returned and saw where the ventilator was set, she screamed that the doctors were trying to kill the baby and had waited for her to go to lunch to lower the pressure. It was a bad scene, with the nurse banging her head hysterically against the wall before things settled down. The mother of the child was not part of any of these events. She was a teenager, unmarried, living in another city, and the only contact the hospital had with her was by phone. The nurse had taken on the role of surrogate mother. Two hours after the ventilator settings were reduced the nurse's "child" died.

Two years later this nurse (as she was moving out of town) went to the district attorney's office and accused Kent Philips of murdering the baby to make room for another baby coming into the nursery. The district attorney took this information to the grand jury. Another nurse, on duty at the time, was called to testify and, to Philips's horror, said that she had seen sicker babies survive. The hospital, also named in the case before the grand jury, decided to defend Philips with, among other things, aggregate statistics. They determined that Philips had the lowest proportion of deaths to admissions and the highest autopsy rate. A review of the baby's chart by other doctors supported the reasonableness of the decision to lower the ventilator setting. After four to five months of deliberation the grand jury decided not to bring an indictment. The total cost of Philips's legal defense came to $12,000, of which $5,000 was paid by the neonatology unit and the rest by Philips himself. He described the experience to me as "hardening." He now covers himself more thoroughly in severe cases by checking with everyone involved with a baby before risking making decisions that might lead to the infant's demise.

March 13. Stephanie is on the special Clinitron bed. She is a very small figure lying on a white, gently rippling background. The air keeping the spheres aloft produces a light and very warm breeze under and on the sides of the sheet placed over the air bed. A strip of cloth loosely seals Stephanie's eyes from the light. Oxygen, white as CO_2 on summer days, drifts up from a tube immediately in front of her nose and mouth. A note of instructions is taped to one of the metal bed posts: "Only one sterile diaper between baby and mattress." Stephanie's mouth is opening and closing slowly, like a fish's jaws long out of water. She yawns, looks satisfied. I am told she threw out her I.V. again last night. Apparently she tenses her abdomen when the nurse works with her.

The Santana baby has beta strep. It is a deadly bacterial infection that can kill full-term babies in twelve hours if not treated in time. He is being given large doses of antibiotics.

Randy Hunter, a Fellow in the nursery, tells me about his experience as a doctor in Madagascar with the Peace Corps. He describes graphically the horror of primitive life, replete with exotic parasites and frequent cases of tetanus. We both agree how truly fragile human life is, and that we live in a society that insulates us from nature and the hostility of the earth to the forms of human life we have in the West. We both scorn the romantic harmony of man and nature eulogized by some traditional philosophers and a few recent enthusiasts in Winnebagos.

It is clear to me that legal discourse has a natural inertia that carries past earlier human experiences into the present. This may help explain why the languages of law currently in use are unable to accommodate the results of recent medical technologies. The neonatal nursery contains new events, unheard of even a decade ago. How can we develop or recognize legal and moral languages to address these new experiences?

From an interview with Peggy Ryan

Frohock: Is it simply the law, then, that keeps people from terminating therapy?

Ryan: Many times, yes. Oh, yes, I think doctors would be much more apt to change their actions. Of course, some of them, I'm sure, would beg to differ with me. When it comes down to brass tacks, I think a lot of them would change their actions if they didn't have Big Brother Government looking over their shoulders, saying, "We're going to get you. We're either going to sue the pants off you and take you for everything you've got or take your license and you'll never be able to practice medicine."

From an interview with Bill Wade. Wade is a careful doctor who is nonetheless admired for his tough decisions on therapy. He is in his mid-forties.

Wade: Set up a theoretical case. For instance, how about a baby born at 400 grams, twenty-four weeks of gestation, who's got a heartbeat of 110 and gasping with expiratory effort. Parents want everything done. Well, everything done and full court press means putting in arterial lines, intubation, ventilation, and a number of other things we can throw in for the child. In the process of explaining to the parents the nonviability of the child, what we generally do is put some of the tubes in but not necessarily hook up the machine. Now we begin to cross a fine line here. It's between lack of intervention and intervention that's been withdrawn. And that gets us very quickly to what most neonatologists worry about sometime in their career—the legalities of what they're doing. The present state of affairs in this country, to my understanding, is that *not* to have committed equipment is okay. It is a different level of magnitude legally than having committed equipment and then withdrawn it. Suppose you don't ventilate a child because you presume nonviability. The evidence for nonviability is very different in that case than ventilating a child and then stopping the ventilator. The ventilator itself, to a lawyer, to the courts, seems to confirm the impression that there was a chance for viability and you withdrew that support. If they die in the face of ventilation no one says anything. Obviously it's a very tough line to draw. To me there's no difference between a child's dying on a ventilator, off of it, or a ventilator not having been committed. It's because of lack of reasonable lung development that the case develops the way it does. There is virtually no difference. The physiology kills them, not the lack of support.

Frohock: Let me explore that thin line for just another minute. Does the fact that it's much more difficult legally to turn off a ventilator than to begin it have an effect on decisions whether to begin it or not?

Wade: Generally not.

Frohock: Why not?

Wade: Well, because most of the babies make the decision for us. If you take a 400-gram fetus, there a foot dragging of ten minutes may be enough. Maybe it's hard to get the machine up. We can do things short of ventilation. You could put a tube

ERRATA

*Through no fault of the author, the text of
this book was printed with the following
errata. These and others will be corrected
in the next printing.*

Page 68, line 14 (missing), should read

arrested in November?

Page 78, line 18 (missing), should read

on therapy entirely to Stephanie's parents
is not enough.

Page 84, line 6

for without affections

read without affectations

Page 108, line 23 (missing), should read

daughter. Do everything for her--always.

in. You could ventilate by hand, for instance, and if there's no significant response with that, you could say to the parents, "Well, look there's no response. Therefore ventilation will not be able to do anything more than we've done by hand-bagging. Therefore, we will not commit this piece of equipment. Okay? But we'll maintain the baby short of that."

Frohock: How about the marginal cases? Cases where one is uncertain but your best guess might be that it's going to be hopeless somewhere down the line. Would the fact that it would be hopeless somewhere down the line *and* the difficulty of withdrawing aggressive therapy once it's begun have a bearing on decisions?

Wade: The tendency there, for most of us, and again I speak mostly for myself and people I have observed—most folks will tend to go for the therapy.

3
Treatment Zones

March 14. Stephanie is in surgery. Her nurse, in sterile attire waiting for her to return, tells me she is "due any minute."

A new baby is in the nursery. His name is Warren Carr. He has no brain. The upper regions of his brain—the cerebrum and cerebral cortex—are missing. Only a brain stem can be verified. It keeps his heart and lungs working. He looks at me and through me. His eyes are at a sunset position, dipping loosely below the skin opening and ready to roll like lemons in a slot machine. His head is enormous, bloated by a concentration of fluid in the skull. One nurse passes him with a "Poor Warren." Another looks at him. "I'm sorry, Warren." There is a slight smell of perfume and sweat in the air. Source unknown.

Warren is the first baby who actually bothers me. There is some aura around him—a grotesque who seems aware of his condition. The nurses talk to him as if there is a self there who, tragically, is missing some vital part of his being. But self-awareness without cognition? This is witchcraft, nonsense. Yet I stand at this moment out in the hall peering in at Warren where he lies at the far back of his room. Is it possible that he and I can suddenly change bodies if I stare one second too long at his eyes? A nurse spies Warren for the first time across the room. "Oh, when did we get him?" Another answers, "This afternoon. From DePaul Hospital" (a local hospital). A third nurse comes over. "They didn't know ahead of time. They did a sonar and it was normal." The first nurse, who is six months pregnant, shakes her head "Oh, no" as she turns away. The nurses are spooked by Warren. But they handle him without any hesitation or signs of revulsion.

These are the most difficult problems in morality that I have ever seen. Is Warren human? Can a creature that can neither see, nor hear, nor think in any way—ever be aware of its environment, least of all its own self—be human?

Warren's treatment will consist of inserting a shunt in his head to drain the excess fluid down to the abdomen. The shunt will be inside the skin all the way down to the abdomen. Once inserted it will not be removed, though it can be adjusted in length as he grows older. There is no further treatment for Warren. He is breathing on his own and is free of infection. A nurse tells me that a baby born like this some time ago went home and lived for a few months before (inevitably) dying. Warren's father, I am told, is in a terrible state of ambivalence, which the nurses relate with macabre humor as a good-news, bad-news story, He is proud to have a boy, but then . . .

Stephanie returns from surgery. She is in good condition. The surgeon found and corrected two intestinal obstructions. Several doctors are in the room with her. It is very hot in there. They need to maintain a high temperature to correct for the loss of warmth through her damaged skin. Stephanie is on a small bed next to the Clinitron bed. The bed has a soft, cottonlike bedding on which has been placed a clean diaper. She is resting on top of the diaper. There are sutures in her abdomen. Bandages of vaseline still cover her ankles and her right wrist and forearm. The nurse says she will be returned to the special bed after she has stabilized from the surgery.

The surgeon's main job was to perform what is called a gastrojejunostomy. This operation hooks the jejunum, which was past the stricture, to the stomach. In this way food goes from the stomach into the jejunum. She tolerated the procedure reasonably well and the doctors expect her surgical incisions to heal.

A mild quarrel suddenly occurs between Stephanie's nurse and an X-ray technician. She won't allow him to move the baby. He finally says with some exasperation, "Then I can't take pictures." After some more conversation they reach a compromise. Stephanie's parents walk in on the tail end of this conversation. They are both in their teens. Neither says a word during the dispute between the technician and the nurse. They watch the X-ray efforts with some interest.

Michael Anthony is awake, his eyes open and blinking rapidly. He seems to be looking at the stethoscope hanging above his head. The respirator tube protrudes from his mouth. He looks like a child sucking on a pacifier who is too old to be doing so. And I suppose the respirator is a kind of pacifier. It keeps this child from the disturbances of death.

The nurses are swapping stories. One tells about a man who brought his wife to the delivery room terrified that he had caused her premature labor contractions by having sex with her the night before. Then story after story follows about women who did bring on full-term labor by having sex in various ways, including the use of vibrators. There is also talk about the use of substances—wintergreen, castor oil—to try to induce labor. It all sounds like bunk to me, except for the parts about sex.

The cafeteria bulletin board is the only permanent sign in the hospital. Every day it announces roast beef at $3.35. And there is never any roast beef.

The two other earlier cases are doing better. Cindy Blackwell is breathing intermittently on her own with the help of a drug. There is still no diagnosis of her condition. Danielle Raymond is doing better each day.

March 14, at night (all night). Stephanie arrests twice during this night. Both times the intern on duty runs down the hall toward her room when the nurse calls on the intercom, his shoes flopping against the floor. He and the nurse work on her each time, adjusting her fluid and medicinal intake and gently shaking her body. One nurse in the hall observes that "she tried to arrest, but couldn't." Another remarks, "She tried, though," as if Stephanie is making efforts to die.

Stephanie's skin is peeling off in places. She is in hell. Why? I have no answer to this question.

At nights the sounds of the nursery are sharper: high-pitched machine whines, gurgling from suction tubes, radio music, ticking (like clocks) of the respirators, elastic snapping and paper diapers being ripped apart as the nurses change the babies, laughter, conversations among the nurses. When the phone rings, the nurses answer "Special care." Then the sounds of therapy: nurses pounding on the backs and chests of babies to clear their tracheal and bronchial tubes. Babies crying. Nurses talking to babies. "Look at you, you're purple" to a baby in oxygen shortage by a nurse reviving him.

In the next room next to Stephanie's isolation unit several nurses are sitting and talking during one of the lulls that seem to occur more frequently at night. One says that she prefers chronic to acute babies, though she doesn't know why. (Chronics are those who are ill for longer periods of time, while acute babies are more intensively ill for shorter periods.) She was drawn to the intensive care nursery because she couldn't handle caring for children who talk, ask questions, link up with her emotionally, and then die. At least, she tells me, the babies here don't understand what happens to them. She is attached to one of twins currently in the nursery. She fought to get him as one of the babies she cares for. She is sitting next to his bed reading on and off. I ask her why she is so attached to him. She looks at the baby. "Oh, he's so stubborn." Apparently he will not go with anyone but her.

Another nurse tells me that the hardest, most stressful event in the nursery is when one of the babies goes into an arrest. "But," she adds, "the most depressing thing is when you do everything for a child and he ends up a nothing. We grow vegetables. Go upstairs to pediatrics and see the vegetables that we grow."

Pediatrics is where the older babies who "graduate" from the nursery are taken. Some are tethered to life-support mechanisms for the rest of their lives, with brains so damaged that they cannot recognize anything. These are the "vegetables." Their graduation from the nursery raises the issue of whether one should keep trying to help some babies. A physician cannot give a verbal command not to resuscitate. He must write out an order—a "no code" instruction—and place it in the baby's medical record. But the nurses say that the doctors will sometimes say, "Go slow on this one."

In Stephanie's room no one is going slow. There is a lot of activity. Two grown-ups are doing everything they can to keep a small creature alive. A technician from the laboratory enters her room with some X-rays of Stephanie. "Everything is normal," he announces. The nurse responds, "Except the baby." Stephanie is still suffering from apnea. Her serum electrolytes and fluid balances have been fluctuating wildly. A short time ago, however, her need for fluids reduced suddenly, resulting in mild congestive heart failure. The intern and nurse are trying to rebalance her electrolytes and fluids and cope with the heart problems. There is some speculation that the heart failures may be related to the increasing area of her body being covered with vaseline. She also may be septic (suffering from a blood-borne infection).

The nursery is organized to treat very ill babies. Nevertheless there are limits to what the staff will do. Occasionally a physician calls from obstetrics, or from a regional hospital, who wants to send over a baby who is well below 500 grams. The doctors in the nursery, with one exception, will stall until the condition of the baby is known with more certainty.

From an interview with Bill Wade.

Wade: The tendency is that if anyone calls for transport, if you can get there to bring the baby back, you go. Even if it doesn't look very hopeful. There are a couple of rare circumstances I can remember where someone would call when the heartbeat was 15 or 20. The baby was an hour, hour-and-a-half old. It was quite obvious that there had been no adequate resuscitation. There was virtually no chance for the child. We asked them to get several more laboratory tests as a way of just letting things settle out, and then call back. It takes about half an hour to forty-five minutes for the transport team to assemble to leave, and so we'll check back. Check back again, and a couple of times it's been so obvious that the team didn't go out. There've been another one or two situations where the child has been so small that we've not been there, 250- or 300-gram child. Obviously well below what anyone can presently try to go for, who still had heartbeat but was making no special effort to survive—a cyanotic kid. The very immature fetuses, lungs aren't developed until about twenty-four to twenty-six weeks—there are virtually no tissues to do anything with anyway. On very small fetuses like that you can just about take the heart out and leave it on the table and it will beat for several hours in that capacity—so it is essentially an extrauterine fetus.

A baby was born recently in the obstetrics wing of Northeastern hospital weighing 440 grams. The doctor on duty in the nursery—Susan Markart in this case—was called down by the obstetrician to examine the child. The baby was vigorous and seemed healthy. Markart brought the baby back up and gave him fluids and kept him warm. She then proceeded to observe the child. After twenty-four hours the baby started to have substantial problems indicating a large intracranial hemorrhage. Markart and the other doctors in attendance decided not to begin aggressive therapy. The baby died in a short time.

The decision Markart made in this case, and the tactics described by Bill Wade, are typical. The physicians in the nursery will not treat babies under 500 grams or twenty-four weeks' gestation unless they continue to breathe spontaneously and maintain a good heart rate. The one exception is Catherine Richmond, head of the unit. She treats everything, I am told. The other doctors feel that under 500-gram, twenty-four-week-gestation babies simply do not have enough air sacs in their lungs to survive. In Markart's words, "You can't ventilate something that doesn't exist." Nor do any of the doctors feel that any foreseeable developments in technology will alter this threshold. Short of inventing an artificial uterus in which babies can continue gestating, 450–500 grams and twenty-four weeks is and will be the lower limits for a reasonable change at survival.

The problem is pulmonary development. The last major organs to develop and mature are the lungs. They do not develop until about twenty-four to twenty-six weeks in gestation. All premature infants have lung problems, some so severe that they will be unable to breathe properly for the rest of their lives. The very small and early babies—those below 500 grams and/or twenty-five weeks' gestation—have little chance to breathe at all even with ventilator support.

All the doctors concede that viability is a tricky term. Some years ago 800 grams was considered the lower threshold of viability. Now, with better skills and technology, it is less than 500 grams. But viability also varies across space as well as time. Babies born close to, or in, a hospital with a tertiary care nursery have a more generous threshold of viability than those born in remote areas distant from high-technology medicine. Even between nurseries there are differences. Individual research interests in hospitals create niches of special care within neonatology itself. If the needed therapy for a baby is extracorporeal membrane oxygenation (cardiac and respiratory support provided by a machine outside the body), for example, then the baby had better be lucky enough to have been born in Virginia or Michigan (the only two states currently carrying out such therapy). Viscosity problems (thick mucus in the lungs or bronchial tubes) are not handled best in these two states, however, for neither has the latest machines to measure viscosity (Northeastern does). Of course, if there are no financial, political, or time problems, babies can be transported to specialized centers. But in the real world there are many impediments to moving babies around from one state to another, not least that the babies themselves do not always tolerate such moves.

Sometimes, the doctors in the nursery claim, the obstetrician sets them up for problems. Some obstetricians administer steroids to pregnant women for certain medical problems, and then will sometimes increase dosages to help prevent stress. The steroids activate the pulmonary surfactant system of the fetus and reduce the risk that hyaline membrane disease will develop. But the babies born prematurely from such women often have severe problems. The nursery physicians admit that without aggressive treatment from obstetricians there would be more fetal deaths. But they are not sure that survival is always preferable. Far more damaging to parents, they argue, is a baby born alive who dies in a few days or weeks, or—even worse—manages to live as a brain-damaged child.

Babies with certain chromosomal abnormalities also are not treated. Trisomy 13 and 18 are the two abnormalities always mentioned. Both cause severe deformity and mental retardation. Children born with these abnormalities usually do not survive beyond the first year of life. Trisomy 21 babies (Down's syndrome) are always treated. Babies with this abnormality are usually retarded mentally and deformed physically. But the variations within the syndrome are wide indeed, ranging from severe mental deficiencies to an intellectual development at which life's events are seen and understood. Also, Down's babies generally lead relatively long and peaceful lives. There is no reason not to treat such children, and all indications are that they are treated, even if parents resist.

One of the difficulties with trisomy 13 and 18 is that conclusive diagnosis can be made only with chromosome tests, and these tests take weeks, not hours or days, to run.

From an interview with Joe Ritiglia, a neonatologist visiting Northeastern. Ritiglia is in his late thirties and has the look of a matinee idol. He is a skilled doctor and is considered the brightest star in his home hospital, DePaul.

Ritiglia: I had a baby who was 900 grams, born at DePaul (hospital) to a family who had had a previous very small premature infant about the same size. This earlier baby had a very long hospital course and ended up with cerebral palsy, but was a much loved member of the family. He is now two, two and a half years old, maybe even older. And the family knew that aggressive therapy made it possible for this child to exist. So this new baby was born at 900 grams and had a number of dysmorphic features that were a little suggestive, but I hadn't put it together a hundred percent. Did fairly well for the first couple of days. Was on a respirator, came off a respirator. Things were really looking up and then one night, just crashed, and this is retrospectively typical of what these kids do. Just absolutely crashed, needed to go back on a respirator, needed tremendous intervention, and during the resuscitation it suddenly hit me what these dysmorphic features were—that this kid was a classic trisomy 18.

So then I had to go up to the mother's room and talk to her and say not only did this baby have a tremendous intracerebral hemorhage clinically with terrible deterioration, but I thought that even at best there was little chance for survival outside the immediate newborn period and no chance of significant intellectual growth. So the parents' response was "Are you sure?" And I said, "I'm pretty sure, but I—you know, in all honesty, I can't tell you I'm positive until I see the chromosomes." And they said "Well, we see what aggressive therapy can do. See here's our baby. We want you to do everything that you can." So, that's what we did. We went along and it lasted for a couple of days. We talked more every day, spent a long time discussing this thing, and they still felt like they needed to do everything that was possible until we knew for sure; and as it turns out, chromosomes take two weeks to get done and though we knew it ultimately, after the baby died, that it was trisomy 18, there was no way that we could tell early on. A lot of parents will go through that. You can make the clinical diagnosis but they want to see the proof.

Babies who are not admitted to the nursery, or who are admitted and then are not treated aggesssively, are dried off, kept warm, sometimes given oxygen (if needed) by a mask placed near the face (but are never intubated or even bagged), and—always—given food in the form of fluids. The rule is to make the baby comfortable while it dies. No starving. No hideous deaths in general. Just a period of tranquil waiting until a heart stops beating that would not have beaten very long, in the doctor's judgment, even with aggressive therapy.

The polar extreme from those cases that are not treated are those that are always treated when the baby is otherwise viable (by far the greater number of cases in the nursery). These include hyaline membrane disease (when occurring in babies beyond 500 grams and/or twenty-four weeks' gestation), meconium aspiration (where the unborn infant has breathed in some of his own feces before birth), hydrocephalus (an abnormal accumulation of cerebrospinal fluid within the ventricles of the brain), trisomy 21, persistent fetal circulation (PFC—the baby's blood is still in a fetal rather than a newborn circulation pattern), intracranial bleeds, and many other serious problems. In this, the larger category, the nursery staff goes all out to save the life of the baby and improve its health.

The most difficult type of case for the nursery is that which falls in the large gray area between do-not-treat and always-treat. Some of these cases are more severe forms of the always-treat variety, or are always-treat conditions occurring in a cluster of problems that makes the baby nonviable. Spina bifida, for example, is almost always treated. But occasionally the nursery gets a baby with a meningomyelocele (hernia of the spinal cord) which is so severe that no one—doctors, parents—wants to treat. (Such seems to be the case of Baby Jane Doe on Long Island.) Other cases are those that a short time ago were do-not-treat and now are ambiguous. For example, a baby born with hypoplastic left heart (the left side of the heart is missing or severely undeveloped) simply died as recently as two years ago. It was a do-not-treat case because nothing could be done to correct the defect. Now surgeons at Northeastern perform surgery on such children. The surgery is a type of bypass that connects the subclavian artery going into the arm with the artery going into the lungs. This shunt allows the intact side of the heart to supply blood to both the lungs and the body. More recently (in July 1984) a three-day-old Dutch baby born with hypoplastic left heart in London was given a heart transplant. She died twenty-five days later of respirator problems. Since the heart was working properly at her death, it is likely that a transplant will be tried again on such babies. But every doctor at Northeastern stressed to the parents the experimental nature of these operations. At the moment the possibility of surgery for hypoplastic left heart has simply made the condition ambiguous, with no one certain whether treatment is warranted or not.

The most difficult cases in this gray zone of treatment are those in which the severity of the medical problem is a variable in locating the baby in either a do-not-treat or an always-treat category. Necrotizing enterocolitis is one such condition. It is a disease in which the bowel of the baby is infected and sections of it die. There is no known cause and the mortality rate is high. Treatment consists of antibiotics, fluids, and general circulatory support. When portions of the bowel die, however, these dead sections must be removed surgically. If sufficient bowel survives, the child can be treated successfully after surgery. This would be an always-treat case. Sometimes, however, too much bowel dies and has to be removed, with the terrible result that the child does not have sufficient intestines to digest food. Such children cannot be fed orally and must receive a form of nourishment called hyperalimentation which is introduced directly into the bloodstream by means of a tube. These children cannot grow into adults and always die, usually from infection, within a few years. The staff at Northeastern treat almost all of these children, but are uncertain whether they should do so, given the inevitable results. Sometimes, however, a surgeon will simply close up a child after discovering the extent of bowel damage. These children die in a few days.

Other cases in the gray area are those babies born with severe brain defects or other terminal diseases for which there are no cures. The anencephalic baby, Warren, is one such baby. Stephanie is another. In both of these cases there is no treatment of the primary problem, nor any plug to pull to allow the baby to die. Warren will probably go home from the hospital in a week or so, there to live a short and unknowing life before dying. Stephanie, at this stage, has a slight statistical chance to survive, though not to be cured of her disease. In the case of Warren, no decision on withholding therapy has to be made. He is living without aggressive therapy, with the exception that a shunt will soon be placed to drain the fluid from his brain. Nor, realistically, is a hard decision on therapy facing the doctors or parents in Stephanie's case at the moment. Having opted for the corrective surgery, the staff now feels obligated to continue their efforts to keep her alive. Like the babies with short-gut problems, not to treat would require withdrawing support that the staff cannot bring themselves to withdraw in cases like this—nourishment and antibiotics. But also like short-gut cases, the doctors are uncertain and even divided over whether treating Stephanie makes any sense.

The zones of treatment decisions, then, are these (with representative cases).

Zone 1 (do-not-treat)   trisomy 13
                                         trisomy 18
                                         under 450 grams and/or
                                             twenty-four weeks'
                                             gestation

Zone 2 (ambiguous)	spina bifida
	anencephalus
	epidermolysis bullosa
	letalis
	necrotizing enterocolitis
	hypoplastic left heart
Zone 3 (always-treat if child is otherwise viable)	hyaline membrane disease
	meconium aspiration
	hydrocephalus
	trisomy 21
	PFC
	intracranial bleeds

If there is a close call in zone 2 the baby usually gets treated.

From an interview with Randy Hunter, one of the Fellows in the nursery. Hunter is an excellent doctor as well as a stand-up comic with a deadpan delivery of outrageous observations. Yet he is humorless when addressing neonatal problems. He also has a medieval reputation for never declining a direct challenge and has been known to engage some of the medical giants at Northeastern in deadly combat.

Hunter: The decision to start aggressive therapy is again one of those that is not—you know you don't spend as much time as some people who have done a fair amount of writing about medical ethics would like to say so. The decision to start aggressive therapy is sometimes made by a person with thirteen months of training in his first couple of weeks of his residency, thirteen months of post–medical school training, in the delivery room with a disaster down there and he doesn't have the benefit of those fancy-pants medical ethicists that want to call committees and come in at two in the afternoon on Thursdays to discuss what the guy, poor slob, should have done down in the delivery room. I mean, he's sitting there sweating his brains out because he has a kid and an obstetrician's screaming and the parents are fainting and he is supposed to be a doctor and taking care of this end and he says—he remembers what Hunter told him on rounds and that is, "If in doubt, if there's ever any doubt, you always, always give the kid the benefit of the doubt and you treat him. If he's going to die anyway, he'll die anyway, but if he's got a chance, you better treat him. Don't let me ever catch you equivocating and not treating a potentially viable kid." So usually they get treated.

Even in the do-not-treat zone, however, parents can mandate treatment, however futile the treatment may be.

From the interview with Randy Hunter.
Hunter: Well, it turns out it's a compromise. You can say you're going to do everything. If a 400-gram premature infant comes out and the parents demand the child be ventilated, well, you can ventilate the kid. If the physician says, "I recommend nothing else be done," you can ventilate the kid, but you don't have to be as aggressive as you would if there was a chance the kid was going to live. Some of it depends on the parents. If it's a term kid with terrible birth asphyxia, but the mother and father have worked with special education kids all their lives and they've adopted two kids with problems— well, we tell them "Look, this kid, this child has had an absolute disastrous course. His kidneys aren't working well. His heart isn't working well. His brain has had a massive insult. There is a chance he will survive—a very, very tiny chance. But if he survives, all the literature we have available now says he's really going to have trouble. Of the ten indicators we have, he has all ten and he's going to be a real neurologic problem." If those parents say, "Look, we've taken care of those kind of kids all our lives, we'll do it," we would go ahead and support that child.

From an interview with Bill Wade.
Wade: One baby, whose meningomyelocele was really high, who had horrible hydrocephalus, had gut problems, terribly disfigured, and probably will never be able to live without a ventilator—the attending physician (who was a neurosurgeon) and I did not want to operate on this baby. The parents insisted that this baby be supported and still be supported despite the fact that nobody wanted to resuscitate this baby if it arrested. [The baby was supported.] So I guess the decision rests with the parents. It also rests with the physicians. It rests partly with the other staff, the nurses, some of the house staff. If the parents want a baby resusci-

tated or treated—the baby will always be resuscitated or treated. If they don't want a baby resuscitated or treated, but the attending physicians and the house staff and the other people who work in the nursery feel that this baby is really ultimately a good baby, that baby may very well be resuscitated. And so I think that the parents sort of have the power to say, "Yes, we always want this baby treated," and I feel always compelled to go with their wishes. Yet, on the other hand, I don't always feel compelled if they say no.

Sometimes the parents do want less treatment for the baby than the doctors think is needed.

From an interview with Susan Markart.

Markart: The last time I was on service, I had a father who was a lawyer. His child was a thirty-two-week gestation baby, which in our hands has a 90 percent plus chance at survival, and of those who survive, 90 percent are perfectly normal children. He said to me, if there's anything wrong with this child, I don't want you to resuscitate. If the baby just doesn't breathe right, well, I don't want you to do anything to my child. This was a big baby. I mean it was twice some of these [in the nursery]. It was a 1500 grammer. And I was prepared. I told him that I will resuscitate your baby. I'll do what I feel is appropriate and then we'll deal with the issues later. In that situation it was just a strong disagreement between the attending physician and the parent. I think there was a lack of education on his part. All he could think of was some premature infant that grows up to be retarded, not normal. He really didn't know how good the baby's chances for survival and doing well were. I think in those cases a parent has to be educated. If you don't have time to do that, you have to do what you feel is right, morally correct. Then you deal with the consequences, whether it be a civil suit and a wrongful life suit. I can deal with that. That doesn't bother me. I've got to live with myself first.

From an interview with Joe Ritiglia.

Frohock: Do you ever have parents from the other direction, who would want to make the error of exclusion? In other words, if there's some abnormality that you feel perhaps warrants aggressive therapy and they feel not—then what happens?

Ritiglia: It hasn't happened yet [to me] but we have had a couple of those cases. I had one mother who had a kid who had a bunch of problems. She kept wanting to know, was this kid going to be retarded? Now it happened that she worked with disabled kids. So she knew what the long-term effects are. But she never wanted to withhold treatment. She never said, don't do it. As it turns out, this was a baby that she was not sure she really wanted initially. She had been thinking beforehand that she might put this kid into foster care or put him up for adoption. She's a very honest, articulate black woman. She said, "I know what my limitations are. I'm young. I'm single. I don't think I could survive taking care of a severely disabled kid." So she was trying to plan for herself. She began to make the emotional separation from her kid. But she was not saying, "Don't do everything that you have to do." And I've never had parents say that. I've had parents wonder, "Should we be doing this? At what point do we call it quits?" That happened recently with a baby. A slightly premature kid who had an overwhelming infection. His mother was a nurse and his father was an obstetrician. As much technology went into this kid as we had to offer. His mother said, "Honestly, at what point do we call it quits?" We kept going through the question, "Well, at what point do we call it quits?" She brought it up. She didn't push it. But she brought it up. We didn't call it quits and, as it turns out, the kid survived and did very well.

From an interview with Randy Hunter.

Hunter: Well, if it's real flagrant, for example if the child comes out with a cleft lip or palate. I've been in the delivery room where a baby was born with a cleft lip and palate. The father said, "My God that's ugly. Don't resuscitate that baby. I'd just as soon that baby die." My first move again is to try to educate him, to try and say, "I know that's shocking. I'm sure you're upset. That's not what you expected. However, something you need to know is that nowadays plastic surgery can repair that very, very well, and the vast majority of these children have everything else normal on them. They have normal intelligence and normal rest of their physical development and normal activity. This is a relatively minor surgical procedure any more compared to the things that can be done. It is a major problem in your eyes. But compared to all the other things that are working so well and that probably will work well, this is really a small problem." If he doesn't go along with that, then I ignore him, because I feel he is so out of bounds. If we're in a gray area of whether it's a middle or high myelomeningocele and a little bit versus a lot of hydrocephalus and that kind of stuff, it's more mushy. Then it takes more sweat and consideration. But in something as simple as that, I will ignore him in the delivery room. If he would physically try and stop me, I would call the guards and throw him out of the door. I would get a court order to have him restrained from killing his child. It would be no different than if a kid came into the emergency room with bad sepsis and the parents say, "We don't believe in antibiotics for this two-year-old. It's against our religion." I would say "That's unfortunate because he's getting it."

The decision not to treat a baby leads to gradual withholding of therapy, and perhaps even overlooking some test indicators or not calling for tests that ordinarily would be made routinely. Some doctors will try to hasten death if a child is going to die in agony over a period of days or even months. But these efforts to hasten death are always acts of omission, in which things that could be done to (in effect) prolong dying are simply omitted.

From an interview with Bill Wade.
Wade: Well, basic chemistry support, fluid, electrolysis management. We may back off on—for instance, if the child happens to be on the ventilator, the decision may be not to increase the settings on the ventilator, not to go to higher pressure, for the child with, say, severe chronic lung disease. Then we'll minimize the number of blood samplings, blood gases, try to reduce the pain inflicted upon the child as much as possible, while still providing nutritional support. Very few families, in my experience, are willing to go the route of not feeding the child something, be it I.V. or be it food. We also will, from time to time for the child who is infected, not add antibiotics, or at least the choice of antibiotics may not be as specific. We may treat with more gentle antibiotics rather than the ones that might be tempered more specifically for that child. That's another way. An error of omission is the word. Most of the infants that have any sort of problem leading to a more prolonged, several weeks long, death, frequently have an

electrolyte disturbance that's part of that. High or low blood potassium, high or low blood calcium, sodium, something that's nutritional, it's cardiac, it's kidney, something with some major organ dysfunction that is going to be affected—that's what they are going to die from, be it early or late. If you don't bother to check those laboratory values, you have nothing to address. If you bother to check and find the potassium is 8 instead of 3½ or 4, you know that—the heart's going to stop. And, if you never bother to check that, there's nothing to correct. You are sort of caught, though, if you do choose to order one of those laboratory tests. Now that you have results, you are now obligated to address those results. And what happens in those situations, we get an intern or resident or somebody who comes through and says, "Well, I ordered electrolytes on everybody in the nursery," and then you find an elevated potassium. Well the next trick of course is repeat the potassium to make sure that it is really high in hopes that you come back with a number that you don't have to address. If you come back with a number you have to address, what you do is short-term therapy, basically. You do something that will correct the value back to normal. Once you demonstrate it's normal, the value will return to the earlier number. And that's not so subtle, perhaps. Then everyone knows what's happening—error of omission, basically. Not addressing what you know is going to be the most likely demise with this sort of child. In terms of acts of commission, I think about the only thing we do from time to time is sedate children with some painkiller, morphine or whatever, that may in some children suppress respiration. It's very difficult to separate the purported therapy from the vehicle [of death] in those cases. In terms of using insulin or potassium or anything else like that as an active thing, there's no way in the world in an intensive care setting that everybody and their brother won't know you've done that. And so that's the impossible thing to do.

From an interview with Joe Ritiglia.

Ritiglia: Really a lot of it depends on parents. Some people will say, "I just can't kill him. I can't withdraw that support that already exists but I don't think he should suffer any more. So if something happens, we should let nature take its course." Then the decision is made not to resuscitate or not to intervene with any further supporting measures. And that can be modified. There comes a point that the family expresses their desires and then the physician sort of interprets. For instance, a kid who's on a moderate amount of support - let's say his lung disease worsens. You can make a decision not to change the respirator. You have a kid who you think has pneumonia on top of it. The usual therapy would be aggressive cultures and intravenous antibiotics. You say, "Well, he's uncomfortable. So we'll make him a little more comfortable. We'll give him some more oxygen. We'll draw some cultures. We'll wait and see whether his cultures are positive." And generally by that time it's too late. So you can do things and you can say, "Well, we did these things." And I think parents seem to deal with that a little better. But it absolutely presupposes that they've been involved in that initial agreement.

And then there are people who say, "You just have to pull the plug. This is terrible. Every second is suffering for this baby. Let's just end it." Now if this happens I would like to encourage the family to be around. Babies generally don't die like that after you pull the plug. They sort of slowly expire. I think to have the family involved at that time is very good. To take the kid off the respirator, to hold him—it may be the first time they've ever held their baby. These kids may go on a respirator on their first day. The parents may never have held their kid and that eats on them after a while if that never happens. To just pull the plug and do it from a distance, it's sort of hard. Getting in close emotionally with the baby, even if it's through the dying process, or even especially, helps them really get in touch and work through their grieving. And that's one of the reasons why a neonatal death is so difficult because they've really not had the chance to establish a good line.

When a baby is not treated, when the case is hopeless, the doctors will move the baby to a special room at the back of the nursery. There, if possible, the parents are allowed to hold their child until it dies. In one case of a child with hypoplastic left heart who also had severe hydrops (the baby's entire body was swollen), the parents decided not to pursue the experimental cardiac surgery. The final moments according to one of the physicians at bedside were "very painful for all involved, but I think it was sensitively done, and it was a very moving thing to see."

3

The cases in the gray zone of therapy decisions (zone 2) present difficult and painful choices for parents and physicians. Especially difficult is recognizing or defining the interests of babies who are suffering from dreadful maladies for which there is no cure and where treatment seems only to prolong suffering. It is in such cases that the anomalies and conflicts of our moral and medical languages seem most clearly revealed

Moral and medical principles are congenial in both of the easy zones (1 and 3) of treatment. If a baby is damaged beyond repair or physical salvation or, conversely, is able to benefit from treatment, the moral and medical imperatives coalesce—either do not treat (zone 1) or treat (zone 3). But the same principles that yield satisfactory outcomes in zones 1 and 3 do not work well in zone 2. The condition of the patients is the problem. Zone 2 babies are damaged in ways that place them at the margins of clear therapy decisions, points at which no one is certain about treatment. Sometimes moral and medical principles conflict in these cases. The right to life of a patient, for example, may mandate treatment in the face of medical judgment that the case is hopeless in the long run. Sometimes morality and medicine are both uncertain guides to therapy decisions, mandating nothing at all. In all zone 2 cases, however, no clear path exists to therapy decisions.

It is worth noting that zone 2 cases are hard even when everyone agrees on the best principles of care. The cases themselves—their complexity, the severity of the problems—allow reasonable people to apply the same principles in different ways. This discretionary power, rather than disagreement on principle, is the main source of disputes over therapy in the gray zone (2) of treatment.

The intern is listening to Stephanie's chest with a stethoscope. He folds the instrument back around his neck. "Lot of junk in there."

The nursery is, finally, a very strange institution. Stephanie's room is a high-stress area, with a doctor and a nurse quietly doing their best with a baby who has virtually no chance at long-term survival. They look at each other from time to time over their antiseptic masks, perspiration dotting their foreheads. Across the hall is a room filled with family-like scenes: nurses feeding babies, burping them, talking playfully to them. Some are rocking their babies to sleep gently in white rocking chairs. In the family room is a baby who has been on a ventilator for one month. He was born with the umbilical cord tightly wound around his throat. The nurses say he is brain-damaged and will never recover. They call him a loser. Then in the next breath they say, you can never be sure. His presence does not disturb the domesticity of the room.

A card in front of one of the rooms: "You have touched me—I have grown." Below the sign is a bulletin board filled with photographs of children who have graduated from the nursery and returned home.

Stephanie is now getting a blood transfusion through a needle attached to her I.V. In the ironic note of the night, a poster on the wall directly across from her room reads: "You're nobody till somebody hugs you." The caption is under a drawing of two bears hugging. The nurse tells me during her break that her fear is touching Stephanie and seeing her disintegrate. Even monitors cannot be attached to Stephanie's skin, and so she must be observed constantly.

The nurses on the night shift knit a lot. One has finished a piece that I cannot recognize when she asks me to guess what it is. I finally say, a lion. No, it is a clam shell.

It is 5:15 A.M. Stephanie seems to be doing better. Everyone is relieved. I offer to make a doughnut run to the all-night cafeteria on the far side of the hospital complex. The run is through tunnels closed at one point by a security door. When the guard asks me through the intercom to say who I am, I answer, "Dr. Frohock" (technically correct). He asks, "What hospital are you associated with?" I cough and say, "Professor Frohock, actually, from the university." He lets me through and I bring back two boxes of doughnuts for the nurses.

At 6:00 A.M. I interview a nurse in the cafeteria room. No tape recorder. I ask her how she feels about Michael Anthony, the six-month-old baby. She answers in a flat tone, "I wish he would die." She thinks it was a mistake to have resuscitated him when he arrested early in his life, though she admits that no one could know then the current extent of his brain damage. She also tells me (in response to a question) that she could never kill to be merciful, though she can only explain this conviction to me by saying that it would be murder. Then she describes an eerie scene. Once, late at night, a baby's ventilator was turned off. The child died shortly afterwards. The nurses kept coming in and out of the child's room while he was dying, looking at him for brief periods of time. It was a strange thing to watch, she tells me, and it bothered the nurses a lot.

March 15 (daytime). Stephanie is recovering this afternoon. Apparently she had septic shock last night. The antibiotics are doing the job today.

Interview today with the dermatologist who is treating Stephanie. At the end of the interview he says, "Doctors are no good. They're not good people." The tape recorder is off at this point of course.

The special care nursery strikes me as a place where decent and dedicated people do and think terrible and wonderful things. The conditions of the place make them what they are, whatever they are. The mysteries in life—birth, death, even sex—are all physically delineated and inspected here. No romance is possible. Matter-of-factness is all. The floating terror here is in having children of one's own. Any number of nurses have related this fear to me. The fear, of course, requires inflating the very small percentage of birth defects to a more generalized norm. I suppose it is easy to take what is a marginal world, a low percentage world, as the norm if you see it continually—if it is your work, your vocation, your reality.

March 16. Stephanie's nurse: "She's doing real well. Better than she should. Than anyone had a right to expect. The book says she should be a lot sicker than she is. Fortunately she didn't read the book." Is it worth it? "It's hard to say. *She's* worth it." How do you mean? "Well, she's got a personality. She's a little human being. And she's doing so well. So I say it's worth it. Now if she should lose her whole skin. Then you have to ask if its worth it to put her through this. It's a day-to-day thing. Today it's worth it."

Warren Carr has a shunt in place, draining fluid from his head to his abdomen. He has started to feed. Doing well, considering his condition.

Cindy Blackwell, the baby with neurological problems, has slept through a spinal tap, which the doctors consider unusual. She is being restrained by straps in her bed because she flails around so much. She is on a respirator. Bill Camisa walks by the crib and fingers the straps. "What are these?" The nurses tell him that they keep her from tossing about. He tells them to remove the straps. "She needs them," they respond. "Take them off." They do so. So far there is no diagnosis of the baby's condition.

Danielle Raymond, the baby born prematurely at a regional hospital, has taken a turn for the worse. She had a slight pneumothorax—the sudden and potentially fatal escape of air from the lungs to the space around the lungs. But she is stable now.

The better-off babies in the nursery are supine, languid—naked reclining figures with just the slightest air of well-being about them. The sicker babies are either restless or in more twisted positions. Their torsos do not look so graceful.

One of the rooms is darkened with the shades drawn. A mother is inside nursing her baby. At last a display of maternal love (I assume).

Susan Markart tells me that they are "into zebras" with the Blackwell baby. A zebra is medical slang at the hospital for exotic diagnoses. It is drawn from the diagnostic rule, "When you hear hoofbeats think of horses not zebras."

A doctor is telling a nurse that he wants a certain baby sent home in a few days. "Let the father touch the kid, smell his poop and urine, love him." A constant refrain among the staff is the isolation of parents from their babies in the nursery. No one knows what the long-term emotional effects of this isolation will be on the babies *and* parents.

Michael Anthony needs almost a regular-sized bed to hold his large and scarred body. He sleeps the sleep of a bank guard after a fight and a celebratory drink. He is sprawled insouciantly across his mattress. There are three teddy bears across his pillow. Attached to the top of his crib is a sign in red letters (a relic from his week in isolation with an infection): "No pregnant personnel."

Jay O'Brien, one of the Fellows, is inspecting a ventilator. "We're going to drown one of these babies with the amount of humidity in these machines."

The full-term baby with beta strep is responding well to antibiotics. He is flushed, confident, a placid expression on his face, sleeping without a trace of a frown.

A husband or lover walks in with green flowers for a nurse. It is St. Patrick's Day. I celebrate with a thoughtless act, accidently walking into a room without a clean white smock. A nurse quickly stops me. "You can't come in like that." I back out with apologies.

Stephanie is back on her special air bed by mid-afternoon. She is crying as the nurse changes her dressings. The nurse tells me that she is regenerating the skin she has lost, which the medical books say she is not supposed to be able to do while still on an I.V. without food taken through the mouth. She won't be able to eat for at least another few weeks. The problem (again) is that her skin sheds from inside her body as well as from outside, and food therefore is a serious irritant as it passes down her esophagus.

What are we seeing here with Stephanie? (1) A baby fighting to live. (2) A look at human feelings at the far edges of extreme pain and helplessness. (3) A game of incompletes: pieces of Stephanie are present while other parts—her skin, her health—are missing. a and b are present, but c and d are not, where a–d is the full complement of an intact human being. Question: Do we get a clearer look at a and b in the absence of c and d? On Stephanie: Do we see *more* or *less* clearly into human suffering when we look at the ravages of her condition, which includes the absence of skin itself? Or would suffering be more accurately displayed in a complete human form?

4
Therapy Decisions

1

The survival rate at the nursery for several years has been in the neighborhood of 90–95 percent. It has dropped a bit in the past two years because more smaller babies and fewer larger babies have been admitted lately. The explanation in both cases is advanced medical skills and technology. The staff at Northeastern more readily admits babies now who are just over or at the roughly 500-gram threshold, and staffs at outlying hospitals are better prepared to treat those babies not so acutely ill (babies that used to be transferred routinely to Northeastern).

Many of the sickest babies in the nursery appeal to the doctors' self-image as crisis managers. Doctors frequently refer to their "wizardry" in medicine and are bored if things are slow (no emergencies). Yet, in spite of the general zest for crises, there is also the brooding presence of uncertainty in almost every decision made. The uncertainty begins with an awareness of the types of mistakes any physician can make. The basic decisions physicians make on therapy are whether to begin aggressive treatment and whether to continue to treat once therapy has begun. The nightmare error is not treating a child who would have survived intact with treatment. Such an error is not easy to detect. As Susan Markart phrased it, decisions of this kind tend to be self-fulfilling ("If a kid is not going to survive, he's not going to survive")—and few postmortems can establish whether the decision or the disease killed the child. Sometimes, to everyone's embarrassment and surprise, a baby survives who has been given up as hopeless. One famous story at the nursery is of a surgeon operating on a baby with severe necrotizing enterocolitis. He judged the disease too far advanced to permit later feeding and closed up the child without removing what he saw as dead intestines. The baby was left to die. But instead of dying he began to improve. Color returned to his cheeks. He began moving vigorously. Every time a staff member looked in on him he seemed better. After twenty-four hours the staff resumed treatment. Today he is at home, a live and vigorous child. Those are the happy mistakes that haunt all of the other decisions on therapy.

Physicians can also err on whether infants need treatment in the first place. Medical therapy is always a trade-off. Benefits are derived from therapy, but all therapy—especially aggressive therapy—has undesirable side effects. A baby can be treated with unneeded therapy that harms or even kills him. Fatalities from therapy are so rare as to be unrecorded. But many on the nursery staff can tell of therapy that was administered poorly, or because of its potent side effects, created problems for the child. In the horror story of the year, one of the babies in the nursery was inadvertently given 17 cc, or three days' worth , of intralipid (a fat emulsion) in an hour and a half by a faulty pump in her I.V. A nurse drawing blood from the baby discovered the mistake when she got a pinkish white fluid instead of blood. (The baby survived.) Such errors seem to be unavoidable, even though Randy Hunter teaches periodic classes on medical errors and how to eliminate them.

The bad effects of even well administered therapy are standard knowledge in medicine. The doctors are currently trying a variety of forms of nourishment for Stephanie: electrolyte water, bolus feedings. All so far have been unsuccessful. She is deficient in calories. So her serum albumin (blood protein) count has fallen to less than 1 (normal is over 3 and even 4). The doctors have treated this by giving her tremendous amounts of amino acids through her I.V. The side effect of such treatment will be that her liver will go through some cholestatic changes and she will develop liver dysfunction and jaundice. Then that will have to be treated. Anyone watching the seemingly endless cycle of treatment, and then treatment of the side effects of treatment, is witnessing a horror show. Mistakenly treating a child who does not need therapy is an error all physicians want to avoid.

The most controversial mistake in the nursery is treating a baby who then lives below some minimal threshold of quality for human life. That such a mistake can be made is acknowledged by all in the nursery, but where the threshold is to be established is a subject of some disagreement. All doctors and nurses can point to some graduates of the nursery who should not have been treated. Extreme cases of brain damage and bodily dysfunction fit everyone's reject list. One child in Pediatrics, Jill Monihan, is a spina bifida victim who has been attached to a respirator for two years and has a brain so damaged that she will never know who she or anyone else is. She also has extensive kidney dysfunction. Her life consists of continual pain from therapy (I.V. and medicinal needles, dialysis, etc.) at a marginal level of consciousness. Doctors regard Jill Monihan as a child who should have been allowed to die some time ago. But since there is great uncertainty of prognosis early on in a child's life, it was very hard at the beginning to say exactly how Jill Monihan would turn out. The doctors are inclined to err on the side of too much rather than too little treatment. *This* mistake is the most common in the nursery.

2

March 17. Michael Anthony is having a six-month birthday party. His parents have driven up from their home in a town fifty-nine miles away. They have brought a cake for everyone and purple and white banners for Michael's crib that say "Happy Birthday." Michael had to be put back on the ventilator (reintubated) today because, according to his nurse, "his whole left side is collapsing." He may need more surgery. His parents are cheerful in a kind of manic way, laughing with the nurses a bit too often. Michael does not, cannot, respond to their sweet talk toward him. The cardiology department made the decision to reintubate. Susan Markhart tells me "They did the right thing. What else could they do?"

Michael's problems are a case study in disaster. He was a full-term baby born with lung problems, a heart condition, and an omphalocele (a hernia of the navel so severe in his case that his stomach was protruding out of the abdomen). He was brought to the nursery the day after he was born in a hospital in his home town. Mary Jane Kennedy, a nurse in Northeastern's nursery, escorted him in the ambulance. His first surgery, performed soon after his arrival, was to repair the omphalocele. It was successful. His heart condition (with the formidable title "tetralogy of Fallot") was improved by two operations, the first to put a shunt in the heart and the second to ligate an extra artery near his heart. He did not tolerate well the anesthetics used in either operation. New problems had been discovered in the first heart surgery. Michael had a hole in his diaphragm (repaired in later surgery) and his liver was found up alongside his heart. Late in his second month of life he suddenly aspirated food into his lungs. It was a full code (complete resuscitation of a patient where cardiac and respiratory functions have stopped). It was at that time that he probably suffered brain damage. His brain waves were grossly abnormal after the episode. He began having seizures and was placed on phenobarbital to control them. At the moment he is taking a number of medications: the phenobarbital, digoxin and quinidine (for his heart), KCL (a potassium additive), Edecrin and Aldactone (diuretics to reduce edema, or swelling). He has not regained consciousness for over three months and he cannot be weaned off the respirator.

Mary Jane Kennedy and I stand to the side of the birthday celebration talking quietly. She is obviously deeply attached to Michael. Why do you love him, I ask. "Oh, because he's getting so old, and he really needs someone. He needs someone to love him and take care of him. He knows me. He knows when I'm here. The other nurses think he's a pain. But how would anyone feel with a tube in your mouth, a sore butt, turned over all the time? Then I think about the kind of life he'll lead and I feel bad. He'll probably be retarded. No one knows how much brain is there. But he's still a human being."

She takes Michael off the respirator tube and picks him up. "Look, Michael. Come on. Do you want to see? It's all right." She places him back on the respirator. "I really thought he was going to die a few weeks ago. He was very unstable. I had two dreams last week that Michael had died. I dreamed I was at the State Hospital and he was covered in blood. But he pulled through." In the dream, I add silently.

Another nurse walks by his crib while his parents are over at the nurse's station. "Bad Michael. Had to be reintubated this morning."

Kennedy counters sharply. "I don't think it was bad that he was reintubated." She shakes her head and looks at me. "It's his birthday. Reintubated on his birthday."

Michael is scheduled for surgery in four days to install a gastrostomy tube so that his mother can feed him (by introducing food through the tube directly into his stomach—a process called gavaging). He is to be sent to a hospital near where his parents live after the tube is inserted.

I ask Kennedy how she will feel after Michael returns to his home town. "Rotten," she answers. "I'll probably be down there a lot. His mom needs a lot of help. She went through a whole grieving period back in November when they told her he was going to die. Now she's finally accepted him. His condition."

She looks directly at me. "What do you think of Michael?"

I look at this large, helpless child. "Well, he's a robust baby." It is the only answer I can think to give.

Stephanie is "holding her own." Her nurse uses a thin tube to suck up the green bile that Stephanie keeps throwing up. So far the staples used as sutures on her surgical incision are holding. No one will venture a guess on how long it will take for the incisions to heal. The nurse says "She's a wild woman today"—tossing about more than usual.

Warren Carr had some minor convulsions during the night, though he is better today. His parents have quietly accepted his condition. His father is a Congregationalist minister.

Cindy Blackwell continues to refuse to breathe on her own. There is talk of doing a brain biopsy if she takes a turn for the worse.

One of the nurses is eight months pregnant. There is a long predictive chart on the wall filled with guesses on the date of birth and weight of the baby.

3

Economists separate decisions according to three types of conditions: certainty, risk, and uncertainty. Suppose that each of a number of alternatives has outcomes. A doctor injects a child with penicillin. The outcomes of the injection can be (a) the bacterial infection from which the child suffers is reduced or eliminated; (b) the penicillin has no effect because the bacteria are a strain resistant to the penicillin; (c) the child has an allergic reaction and becomes seriously ill and perhaps dies. In conditions of certainty the doctor could say with assurance which outcome will occur. Conditions of risk state that the doctor can attach reasonable probabilities to the outcomes. Uncertainty conditions mean that the doctor cannot even say with assurance what the probabilities are.

There are certainties in medicine. The physician who injects a child with a large dose of potassium at any time of the day or night knows without any doubt that the child will shortly die. But positive therapy almost always falls somewhere between risk and uncertainty. Rough probabilities can usually be assigned to a variety of possible outcomes on the basis of clinical evidence and previous experiences, though sometimes even probabilities cannot be reasonably constructed. At all times the staff is seeking additional evidence in order to increase, however slightly, the reasonableness of diagnosis and treatment.

Even clear-cut cases may turn out to be other than they appear.

From an interview with Randy Hunter.

Frohock: Would you resuscitate Warren Carr?

Hunter: If someone called me out on to the nursery right now and said "The baby's arresting, what should we do?" there would be no hesitation in my voice; with the information that I have, I would say resuscitate him. And I will resuscitate him if no one else will, because I don't have the information. The next thing to do would be to collect data, in fact see if there's any brain there. He wouldn't be the first child that was sent to us and they said he had no brain and, in fact, he did. He just had a thin cortex squashed by hydrocephalus. Once that was drained, the child perked up and did reasonably well. You need to carefully collect your data and make sure your information is right. It's rather a major decision for this child. If in fact I had that data in hand, that the child only had brain stem function and therefore would be devoid of all intellect, vision, hearing, emotion, and the truth of the matter is would not survive long-term—I mean they just don't survive long-term even when they're treated—then that child, once all that data was collected and that information was solid and reviewed by competent people, the radiologist who had experience with children CAT scan, that kind of stuff, then, in fact, I could with a good conscience not resuscitate.

Collect and review data—this is what doctors do again and again, continually updating information on a child. A physician approaches a case like a policeman trying to solve a homicide. He uses instinct, training, experience, colleagues, and is a bear for information. Unlike the policeman, however, the physician is always constrained by time—he has to make decisions quickly on occasion, and without adequate information.

Decisions made very early in a child's life are less reliable than those made later when additional hypotheses are confirmed or falsified. One problem early on is that information (such as chromosome tests) may not be available yet. Another, more serious, problem is that very young babies have not developed enough for physicians to say with reasonable assurance how grave their problems are. The earliest decision is whether to treat a baby at all. This is a time of great importance and poor prognostic certainty. Is the infant viable? What is the likely outcome of the baby's condition if she lives? Is there time to run more tests, let things develop a bit before making a commitment?

The pattern that seems to characterize early decisions in the gray zone of treatment is one of incremental moves with a gradually increasing number of people being consulted. (1)The first move, unless there is an emergency (and the doctors at Northeastern tend to apply massive therapy if facing a life-or-death decision without information), is to stabilize the child in order to (a) wait and see how the patient progresses and responds to routine therapy, and (b) secure additional data that might make diagnosis more reliable. (2) The second move, following immediately on the first, is to consult with colleagues, relevant specialists, and the child's parents. (3) Treatment continues along with constant evaluation of the patient's capacity to benefit from treatment, followed by (4), either a change in the patient's condition (to worse or better) that mandates a decision in clear and indisputable ways for the attending physician, *or* a continuation of uncertainty in which nevertheless the physician decides either not to be heroic if an arrest occurs, or to begin aggressive therapy with the aim of saving the patient. Most decisions, according to doctors, do not have to be made. The child declares himself one way or the other (makes the decision for the doctor by taking a dramatic turn for the worse and dying, or by showing signs of improvement that clearly justify aggressive therapy).

From an interview with Randy Hunter.

Hunter: The way he [a colleague] does it and the way I try and do it is that they [the parents] are always a part of the decision. You never just make that decision without their input. When the difficult decision comes up, you collect data as best you can. You formulate a plan and get things pretty much settled in your mind. And, of course, that's ten minutes' work there. It would be wonderful to have five days. But you don't have five days. You have ten minutes while the nurse is bagging the baby [administering oxygen manually] to decide whether to put the kid on the ventilator or not. You go to the parents in less than optimal circumstances, which is that they're still in shock because the Gerber baby they thought they were going to have comes out and has all these problems. You try and give them the basic outline of information and as informed an opinion as possible. It's less than optimal. It's not what you would like it to be but that's unfortunately the way life is right now. I mean, you don't have five days and a committee to call. You often have just a few minutes. So you need to sit down with the parents, talk to them, try to get an idea of what they feel, how they react to the situation. And when they ask you for your opinion, you tell them your opinion as honestly as you can. How do I approach it? I take care of the kids like they were my own kids. I just tell them, here's the way I think, here are my feelings. If it were my own child, this is how I would do it. Because there is no child I would care for more dearly than my own and if I were doing it, that's how I would do it.

From an interview with Joe Ritiglia.

Frohock: Which is the harder decision for the doctor—deciding to begin therapy, or to stop it?

Ritiglia: Well, I don't know what you mean by harder. Starting therapy—it's easy. You don't have to make decisions. You just do it. And it covers you. That's not necessarily to be completely negative about it. It gives you the opportunity to spend some more time to really think out what you want to do. So it's sort of a continuum. It's not really two separate issues. Occasionally the decision not to institute treatment is clear-cut. More often than not, it's not clear-cut and it's much easier to just go ahead with routine intervention—which may be drastic, but in this business drastic intervention is routine. It's much easier to just proceed with that and then get everybody together.

We're assuming that there is a decision to be made. I'm presupposing that you're dealing with either a very tiny premature infant or a baby who has the potential for being severely brain-damaged or something like that—that's the only time that there is a problem. The decision, in order for it to be a good one, has to be one which is made under optimum conditions: least emotional tumulut, greatest information and maximum participation of all people involved. I'm not saying that you can get all those things. But to make the best decision, those things need to be accomplished. That's frequently not the case at the outset of a baby's life, no matter how difficult or no matter how involved medically the baby happens to be. So it's nice to be able to institute something just to stabilize the situation—to group all the parties around you, provide whatever information you can, deal with things emotionally, get over the initial shock, and then help people make a decision as to what they want to do. Sometimes there's no decision to be made after that. If the baby is, for whatever reason, obviously in a tenuous state to begin with, it may well have made such a dramatic improvement that there's no longer a decision. That happens in a pretty significant number of cases.

Early decisions on therapy seem free of several of the constraints found in later decisions. Many are simply acts of omission. Whether clear and consistent distinctions can be drawn between acts of omission and commission is itself uncertain. But the doctors are aware of the *legal* differences between witholding therapy and withdrawing therapy once it has been started. Early decisions are also not bound by previous commitments of medical resources. The slate is still clean. There is no *history* of decisions. There are also, early on, relatively few people who might affect the decision. Consultations widen dramatically later, but at the beginning the group of medical personnel is small.

Later decisions, especially those involving continuation of aggressive therapy, are less autonomous. They are constrained by the inertia of past decisions and the law. Doctors hate to admit they have been wrong, and withdrawing therapy is such an admission. Also, withdrawing therapy, especially ventilators, seems too much like direct killing in the eyes of some doctors, nurses, and district attorneys. Each of the medical figures involved in the decisions has a special interest in saving the patient. One nurse argues that no physician sees all of Michael Anthony. Different teams of doctors look at him—pediatrics, pediatric surgery, cardiology, neonatology. Each team is inclined to go all out to maintain their part of his body. Nurses, she says, are the only ones who see the whole child all of the time. Parents also are constraints on later therapy decisions. They become much more attached to children as time passes (though—and this is clear from interviews—the attachment is both positive and negative). Finally, nurses become emotionally attached to babies over time, an attachment more nearly supportive than that which many of the parents can muster. Michael Anthony's parents are typical. They are bonded to him, but cannot stand to see him too frequently. Everyone tells of the parents of another severely damaged child who appear at the hospital only when he arrests. They weep and demand that everything be done to save their child, but then disappear until the next arrest. In a later decision, the greater number of people involved and the richer emotional context are both restrictions on what the physicians can do. The irony is that later decisions are often accompanied by much greater prognostic certainty.

March 19. Stephanie, according to her nurse, is doing "as well as could be expected" (surely the great medical cliché of this and all other years). The nurse says "She's got the wiggles today. Almost wiggled off her bed." Her I.V. tubes are wearing out. But no one wants to try to insert new ones yet, given her skin problems. So she struggles along with her lifelines in shabby shape. Her personality still attracts. The nurse tells me, "She pouts a lot. She's really something." The sutures on her abdomen look like metallic coils.

The baby with beta strep is nearly well. He is awake, glancing around (it seems) at his surroundings. He is, as a healthy baby, an obvious anomaly in this setting. Now he is crying lustily as his diaper is changed. What a great sound!

Cindy Blackwell is still on the respirator. Eyes staring blankly.

One survivor of twins is lying quietly in her bed. She couldn't be more than 600 grams. Her face is swathed in bandages. Again I ask myself the question—Do such tiny beginning creatures die, or simply fail to live? Perhaps I am not phrasing this question right yet, for nothing remotely resembling an answer comes to mind. A technician is applying a sonar test to the baby's head to check for intracranial bleeds. The instrument, which looks like a hair dryer, is placed on a vaseline-greased section of the scalp. A black and white TV image appears on a screen. Gently moving the instrument shifts the images. I ask whether the instrument is accurate. No answer. Finally, after my third attempt, the technician says that it is. Then she adds that it is better than a CAT scan in one important respect: the test can be run on the baby without moving him from his bed.

Michael Anthony is breathing on a respirator. He is an earthbound astronaut tethered by his mouth to a black rubber tube. There is a smell of alcohol around the bed. The "Happy Birthday" banners are still hanging from the top part of his crib. A nurse tells me she is dubious that he will be moved to his home town since he is still on a ventilator.

March 20. Stephanie's nurse is talking about stress. She says that the fetuses of women under stress develop more rapidly. I ask her what makes some babies fighters and others not. "It's hard to say. Some 500-grammers come out screaming and kicking—you just know they're going to make it." Would you have treated Stephanie at the beginning? "You really have to. Yes, I would have. Because you never really know. She's surprised everyone. I was here when the O.B. came in. He just came in without any sterile protection on, just his street clothes. He said, 'Well, you know, these babies never make it, so it doesn't matter.'"

Warren looks better. The shunt is working. His head is down to almost normal size. He is not eating well yet. One of the nurses in his room wants to go home early. "I've been here eleven hours." She is told she can't leave. She affects a mock frown: "We can leave all of the babies an automatic pilot." Warren is rolling his eyes while sucking on a bottle. He is endearing—there is no other word for it.

Stephanie's nurse tells me that she is pooping. I ask if that is a good sign. "Yes, it show her systems are starting to work."

The local hospital is ready for Michael Anthony. The doctors in the nursery are overjoyed. One actually shakes Susan Markart's hand (she has arranged the transfer): "You are a champion." Several doctors, though, can't quite believe Michael will be transferred and question Susan about the certainty of the move. "Will it really happen?" one asks.

The phone rings. It is Mrs. Anthony, Michael's mother. Mary Jane Kennedy talks to her. "I know, maybe I can come down and visit him. Just make sure they let me in. I don't want to see him through a window. I'm going to miss him, I don't even want to think about it. I have this picture on my makeup mirror. I see it every morning. Do you have a piece of paper? Why don't I give you my number. Okay. Yeah, take care." Michael is now hooked up to the latest machine in the nursery—a multisystem space lab monitor (or so it seems) that can show heart and lung rates at the same time and superimpose them on traces of the rates from previous moments. He is at this moment displaying periodic trigeminy (two normal heart beats in a row followed by a skipped beat).

From an interview with Mary Jane Kennedy. Kennedy is a person who forms deep and lasting attachments to those she cares for. She jealously protects "her" babies in the nursery.

Frohock: How did you get into nursing?

Kennedy: Believe it or not, I was in the third grade.

Frohock: You became a nurse in the third grade?

Kennedy: (*Laughter*) When you're in third grade, when your teacher asks you to write your paper on what you want to be, I just wanted to be in nursing. Ever since then. Nobody in my family has been in medicine. I just wanted to be a nurse and that's the direction I went.

Frohock: What do you like about neonatal care the most?

Kennedy: The kids. I just get a real satisfaction out of them. I enjoy working with them. A lot of people say it's different if you have your own kids. I can see that. I don't have kids to go home and take care of. The kids here occupy my mind, even when I am out of here.

Frohock: How long have you been in the unit?

Kennedy: Two years in June.

Frohock: The first day I was up here I learned about the distinction between acute and chronic children and everyone told me some nurses prefer acute and some prefer chronic. Do you have any preferences?

Kennedy: I don't choose chronic children. I usually take them in their acute stages and they just turn out that way. I don't plan on them to be chronic but that's how a lot of them end up being—especially cardiac kids. I never dreamed in a million years that I'd like a cardiac kid, but it seems the past three babies I have cared for in two years have been cardiac kids. They are babies that have been here for a very long time, over four or five months.

Frohock: How long have you cared for Michael Anthony?

Kennedy: Michael was born the day before my birthday in September. He was transported here on my birthday. I cared for him then for two months. He had a very bad arrest in November. I couldn't even look at him for a few days after he arrested. He was so out of it. He looked horrendous to me. I just couldn't take care of him for a good month. It was right after Christmas that I picked back up on him. I don't know what it was. I couldn't believe he actually arrested and was not alive for a half an hour and they brought him back. I knew something had to have gone on in his head—for him to have been so hypoxic for a half-hour. It was right before Christmas that I picked him back up. He had one of his collaterals tied off and I went to surgery with him. I remember in surgery he had a very bad arrthymia. His surgeon, a very good surgeon, couldn't believe that Michael could have such a bad arrhythmia. He was very upset and he is a wonderful doctor. When I saw how upset he was in going to operate on Michael—that's when I think I started getting very attached to Michael. A lot of people didn't have confidence in Michael. He needed some strong support behind him, and that's where I thought I could really be behind him, work with him. I went away after that to Boston. I remember calling home the next day to see how he was. I think that's where Michael and I got tied back up again.

Frohock: I want to ask you a very hard question. Would it have been better not to have resuscitated Michael back when he *arrested in November?*

Kennedy: Probably. It would probably be better off for his parents if they hadn't. As much as I love him, I think we put that kid through hell here. The pain he's gone through. Yes, we celebrated. I had that big six-month birthday party for him. Six months of hurt. He never has known anything else. All he knows are the words I give him and the cuddling I give him. That's the only nice things he knows. He doesn't know what it's like to play in a playpen or—he just lays there. We've really tortured him. I don't want Michael to die. He's been through all this—I don't think I could sit in on an arrest with him. I don't think I could. I would have to walk away and have everybody else do it. I look at him and I think, "What am I doing to him? Am I prolonging all his agony?" I think that's just what we all did to him. He has a very bad prognosis. Are we keeping him alive for a couple of days, for a couple more months? Is this all going to end?

Frohock: What do people think about when they try to resuscitate a child like that? Do they ever consider not doing it?

Kennedy: No, we never can.

Frohock: Why not?

Kennedy: It's our job. We have to. It's the law. It's the law. It's a sick law, I think, because it's so easy to make a law and say "You've got to keep that baby alive." All those people that are making these laws—do they take these kids home? Look at all the parents. What about those parents that take some of these kids home that just lay in their bed? Then that doesn't even—the financial problems. Can you imagine what Michael's medical bills are right now?

The pit-stop baby recovering from beta strep has a green card hanging in his crib. It reads:

> Dear Mr. Patrolman—
> I am not drunk
> My state of confusion
> is caused by a magic spell
> cast over me by
> a green spotted leprechaun
> that I met while trying
> to drive the purple snakes
> out of Joe's bar
> Please point me toward home which is at:
> and the top of the evenin' to ye and ye'rs.

One of the happy and successful graduates of the nursery has returned for a triumphal visit. A small boy, four years old, makes the rounds of the rooms with only a slight limp. The nurses fuss over him with genuine delight. His parents are at some point beyond pride—they are ecstatic and overjoyed. It is a happy scene.

March 21. Stephanie is doing poorly. She has a low rectal temperature, poor heart rate. Rebecca Smith is her nurse this morning. I ask her: Would you have treated her at the beginning? Long pause. "Yeah, you have to. If she were mine—here you have a baby who's neurologically intact. She's fierce. You can tell which of them is going to fight. Some give up. I've seen the chronics just give up. She hasn't. She's fighting. The life she'll lead. The dermatologist said this morning that he had one like this as a patient. She couldn't even put on a pair of socks when she got older. So should we put her through all of that? I'm just glad I don't have to make the decisions." Is she suffering? "I've seen adults with G-tubes and everything in them who are afraid, who think their condition is gross. Babies of this age don't know these tubes and so on are gross. So they don't have that suffering—mental agony. She's suffering physically, but at least she's spared the mental agony—and that's a lot of it."

In the most intensive wing of the nursery several doctors are rushing down the hall. What's happening? One turns quickly to me. "Baby Raymond is crapping out on us." I follow this doctor into room B. Danielle Raymond's bed is surrounded by doctors and nurses. Bill Camisa is trying to see if the intubation line is in her tracheal opening. A nurse tells me that Danielle's heart rate went down dramatically a short time ago. They have already injected her with a heart stimulant. The baby is gasping in what is surely a terminal agony, her arms reaching up in slow motion to grasp something. A nurse implores here quietly, "Come on, sweetheart." Bill Camisa shakes his head in disbelief, "I don't believe my eyes. I swear there's another tracheal opening down there." An X-ray technician arrives with his large machine making its warning sounds. He takes an X-ray of Danielle. A nurse kisses the baby on her stomach. "Danielle, you're so cold, sweetheart." An intern listens with a stethoscope to the baby's chest. "There's a good heart beat." A nurse comments, "Yes, drug-induced." Danielle in languid poses, bony chest heaving spasmodically, arms thrown across ventiltor tubes. The same nurse kisses Danielle several more times. "What did the X-ray show?" Camisa squints at the negative held up to the light. "Either a total collapse of her lung, or fluid—not good." Another nurse says that Danielle "looks terrible." The nurse who has kissed the baby disagrees. "No, she looks better." Bill Camisa examines her. "Whatever the density is, the drug helped."

In the midst of this activity, Danielle's mother unaccountably calls. An intern talks to her. He explains in considerably less dramatic tones what Danielle's condition is. The mother asks if the baby can eat soon. Background guffawing when the interns repeats the question aloud. He holds his hand over the phone, then replies in calm voice, "No, we don't expect that soon. It's a matter of seeing what's happening."

A nurse stomps her foot impatiently as Danielle's heart starts to beat erratically again. She caresses the baby's arm and chest. "Come on, Danielle."

After twenty minutes more of waiting, Danielle Raymond is stabilized. Her heart and respiration are back to normal. Danielle is ten days old today.

Across from room B is a room with a white shade drawn across the window. A sign on the door says, "Mother nursing." This is the same room in which the fetus was left to die last weekend.

This is Michael Anthony's day for surgery to install his feeding tube. He is due in the operating room right away. Mary Jane Kennedy is in a frenzy of irritation. "No way will he be ready." Michael is staring blankly, blinking, arms apart, huge chest and stomach thrust out. He is a barroom fighter who has gone a bit punchy but is still formidable for a round or two. The transport for Michael arrives. It is a square mobile bed with a bottle of compressed air hanging from its side. The nurse bringing it instructs Mary Jane on how to work the oxygen supply. Michael has a bright red dinosaur on his bed. It is a birthday present from his grandmother. Kennedy suctions out his nose and throat for the last time before leaving. "I think we've got everything, babe." The word "girth" is pasted on Michael's stomach, indicating to nurses where exactly to measure his bulk. Kennedy disappears. She returns, her face freshly powdered. She and the other nurse take Michael to the transport bed. He craps in his diaper as he is deposited on the bed. Kennedy yelps in disgust. "Aiee. When did you do that?" The other nurse says, "It looks like he had spaghetti for dinner." Michael is oblivious. He's back on an oxygen tube from the hand-driven portable ventilator. The nurses quickly and efficiently clean him up. Michael leaves for the operating room with three nurses escorting him and covered with white clothes. At last he looks cuddly. The entourage pauses at the elevator to check Michael's pulse. No one can find it in the confusion. Everyone is laughing except Michael. Kennedy runs over to push the halt button on the elevator. "We're going to stop this fucker until we're ready." At last the group gets on the elevator and the doors close. Bon voyage, Michael.

Kennedy returns in a short time. Her mood is reflective. "Michael likes Diana Ross. She was singing when he left for his last surgery. And she was singing when he came back three hours later."

Warren Carr is squinting and blinking at his own hand. The nurse comes over. "He's doing better. Poor thing. But it may not be as bad as they think because he's eating. Babies with big heads usually don't eat. He's badly off. But not as bad as poor Brian there, who is severely retarded." Brian is on a ventilator. He is the baby born with his umbilical cord twisted with two knots around his neck. His brain is badly damaged. He will eventually go home when he gets off the ventilator. His mother will have to suction him frequently. She is seventeen years old. There is enough work with this child to keep her fully occupied for the rest of her life.

A monitor on a baby shows a flat line (indicating no heart beat). The nurse flips the monitor off. "The baby looks all right. It must be the machine." Appearances can be decisive in the nursery. Nurses will again and again let their observations override technology.

The baby with beta strep is now fully recovered. He is being fed in the level 2 wing. He looks good. The nurse smiles sweetly. "He was circumcised last night. He didn't like it."

Cindy Blackwell continues to perplex the doctors. No diagnosis. She is lying quietly in bed hugging her respirator line.

Stephanie is scheduled for surgery this afternoon to replace her I.V. line. The problem is locating another area on her body that will take and hold the line. Her parents are here. They are a young, sturdy couple appearing to be in splendid shape. They are irritated that they have not been able to see the dermatologist treating Stephanie. Stephanie is particularly lovely today. She really *can* capture your affections if you spend time around her.

A cleaning woman is scraping up tracks of feces from the floor with a mop. Bill Camisa grabs my arm and announces that Danielle Raymond is "stable as a rock now."

"Stairway to Heaven" is playing on the radio. In the background is the steady whine of breathing monitors. It is a moment when one asks, What kind of a place is this? "Time in a Bottle" begins playing. A special type of person is found working in special care nurseries. One is reminded of the line in the movie *All That Jazz*—"On the wire is life. The rest is waiting." What kind of person thrives from being on the wire continually?

From an interview with Mary Jane Kennedy

Frohock: What's the toughest part of your job?

Kennedy: The stress. The intensive care stress up here. There are days that you go home from here so totally exhausted you can't move. And not just physically—mentally. Especially when you have such an acute kid that you're taking care of and you've got fifty doctors around you saying to do this, do that. Every doctor's giving you a different order and you don't know where your head's at. Then with Michael—he had a cardiologist and he had surgeons and he had our doctors. When you get an order from each one of those different services, your head is spinning. Wait a minute, cardiology just told me to do this, and now surgery's telling me to do this? It's completely opposite. Sometimes it just doesn't make sense.

Frohock: So what do you do to unwind? How do you get away from the stress part of it and survive?

Kennedy: Go home, sit in front of the TV. Go home, exercise. Exercise seems to be the best. Go and work out, or just sit home and do some needlepoint or needlework or . . .

Frohock: I want you to tell me what is the best thing you've seen since you've been working here, and the worst thing.

Kennedy: Okay. The best thing was Michael. He's the best thing that's been here, probably, to me. Worst thing? I had another baby that died last February. She went through cardiac surgery. I stayed with her parents. They were from out of state. I stayed with her parents all day during surgery, finally went home at midnight. The parents called me at 5:00 A.M. to come back because Mary Ann had died. I came in and saw her and I just never believed it was the same baby that I cared for for five months. She was—she just, after her surgery and after them trying to resuscitate her, was just a mess. I'll never forget that in my mind. She was just a big puff ball about five times her size.

5
Life and the Quality of Life

Modern social theory provides a generic definition of rationality. One is rational if one selects alternatives that realize one's interests. Sometimes these interests are said to extend to others. Sometimes they are seen as more narrowly egoistic. The rules to follow in selecting alternatives do not have a generic expression. Decision theory has taught us that what it is to be rational will change with the conditions in which we find ourselves. Different rules are rational in different circumstances, a point made at great length in many learned works. Nowhere in social theory, however, do we find a full account of what it means to be rational on behalf of another.

The social theorist may find it interesting then that decisions on therapy in a neonatal setting are always representational. They are made on behalf of patients who cannot, because of their age (whatever their condition), make decisions for themselves. Physicians are rational when they try to secure the interests of their patients (of whatever age) in life and health. Sometimes these interests are difficult to fix, even when the patient tries to express them. But the neonatologist, unlike most other specialists, can *never* ask his patient to help in recognizing these interests. The individuals at the center of neonatal medicine are infants, who, by definition, must be represented by those who can be rational in their interests.

Settling on the interests of very young babies seems impossible at times to the neonatal staff. The most difficult issues of interest are produced by the success of physicians in keeping babies alive who are suffering from dreadful maladies. The case of Stephanie is a powerful illustration of this dilemma. She is suffering from a disease for which there is no cure. The mortality rate is in the 99 percent range. At the moment her doctors are virtually certain that she will not survive the illness much longer. If she lives, her life will be one of daily pain and constant vulnerability to disease. The treatment itself causes suffering, as does any touch of her body. Treatment continues, though no one believes it will restore her to health or save her life.

What are Stephanie's interests? It is easy to say that she wants to live and would express that interest if she were able to do so. But would she want to continue living in her present condition with the prospects at hand? An interesting case occurred at the time of Stephanie's treatment. In the winter of 1983 an elderly man in Syracuse, New York, began starving himself in a private nursing home. The eighty-five year-old man began to refuse food on December 21 after a stroke left him unable to walk unaided. The man, G. Ross Henninger, had been a prominent electrical engineer and president of Ohio Mechanics Institute, and had served as United States trade representative on technological matters to France and India. At the time of his fast he had been confined to a wheelchair for months and was suffering from heart disease, arthritis, and hardening of the arteries. Mr. Henninger told his doctor that he wanted to die.

The nursing home reported the fast to local authorities and asked a judge to clarify its rights and responsibilities to Mr. Henninger. By this time Mr. Henninger had lost 40 pounds and was obviously serious about carrying out his intentions. After hearing testimony on his competence, the judge ruled that the nursing home was neither obligated nor empowered to force-feed him. Two days later—forty-five days after beginning his fast—G. Ross Henninger died. Friends and family described his life as full, using words like "intense," "committed," "energy and ambition." After his stroke, his daughter said, "He couldn't control his hands enough to control any kind of machinery. . . . He couldn't read anything significant." At the end of a long and full life, Mr. Henninger decided—rationally, competently—that these debilities made his life not worth living.

Discussion of Henninger's case was predictably divided in the days following his death. The local Right to Life Foundation viewed the court decision as a frightening precedent. They saw it as analagous to allowing someone to jump off a bridge. The American Civil Liberties Union, however, viewed the case as an endorsement of an individual's right to privacy, to choose how and under what conditions he would live or die. The key to the court decision was the ruling that Henninger was competent. Also, he was deciding for himself, able by means of his own efforts to carry out his wishes, and was not in the custody of the state. Several parallel cases illustrate how courts rule when those criteria are not found. On the day that Henninger died, a judge in New Jersey appointed a guardian to decide on treatment for a frostbite victim who had refused the partial amputation of his feet urged by doctors as needed to save his life. The man, who claimed God would take care of him, was judged mentally incompetent. In an earlier case, an appellate court in Rochester, New York, ordered a state psychiatric hospital to force-feed Mark David Chapman, John Lennon's assassin, when he was on a hunger strike. The decision was based on the state's obligation to care for prisoners in its custody. The New York State Court of Appeals, in yet another case, did not allow a competent parent to make a right-to-die claim on behalf of his incompetent child.

The courts are not consistent on the criteria of individual competence and capability. At the time that Henninger died, Elizabeth Bouvia, a mentally competent quadriplegic in California, was not allowed to starve herself in a hospital. The court ordered the hospital to force-feed her on the grounds that Ms. Bouvia's right to take her own life did not compel the hospital staff to stand by while she starved. It appears that mental competence, acting for oneself and not for others, and not being a ward of the state are legal conditions for suicide only if one is in New York rather than California.

The differences between Henninger and Stephanie are instructive. Stephanie is not—obviously—able to make any decisions or carry out any action. Judges have ruled, in the case of comatose patients, that decisions on maintaining life-support therapy can be made on the basis of substituted judgment—what an individual would decide were he able to make such a decision. Often the evidence used in the construction of such hypothetical decisions includes written documents ("living wills") in which the individual sets out the terms in which he would prefer death to life. Twenty-two states and the District of Columbia now legally recognize such wills. In one case, *Matter of Eichner*, both the Appellate Court (1980) and the Court of Appeals of New York (1981) accepted reports of oral intentions. An eighty-three-year-old priest, Brother Joseph Fox, suffered a cardiac arrest during hernia surgery that left him with substantial brain damage. He was described without challenge in the court as in "a vegetative state." One of his colleagues in the order, Father Eichner, petitioned to turn off Brother Fox's respirator. Since Brother Fox had said on two earlier occasions that he would not want his life prolonged if his condition were hopeless, the court allowed Father Eichner to express Brother Fox's wishes in substituted judgment. Both courts held that the respirator could be turned off.

The problem is that Stephanie has led no life, and so no evidence of any kind (written or oral) can be provided for how she would decide her fate. Someone else must decide for her. Two other court cases offer better parallels. One is the famous Karen Ann Quinlan case. In this case the parents of a nineteen-year-old New Jersey girl who was in a vegetative coma asked the hospital to disconnect her from her respirator. The court (1976) acceded to the parent's request (whereupon, to the doctors' surprise—though not to that of the nursing staff, which had slowly been reducing Ms. Quinlan's dependence on the respirator—Ms. Quinlan proceeded to breathe on her own). In a more recent case, *Matter of Storar*, the appellate court permitted the mother of a terminally ill and profoundly retarded adult to halt blood transfusions for her son. The court held that "a person has a right to determine what will be done with his own body and, when he is incompetent, this right may be exercised by another on his own behalf." However, this order was reversed on appeal. The appeals court (1981) held that an incompetent patient should not be allowed "to bleed to death because someone, even someone as close as a parent or sibling, feels that this is best for someone with an incurable disease." Rather, the *evidence* on the case should be inspected. And, since the transfusions did not involve excessive pain for Storar and they allowed him to maintain his mental and physical abilities at their usual level, the court ruled that they should have been continued.

The most recent *Storar* ruling, in contrast to the *Quinlan* case, does not allow parents to be the uncontested surrogates of their children. Indeed, on the *Storar* holding, the merits of a case are more important than representation on issues of life-sustaining treatment. A New Jersey Supreme Court ruling in January of 1985 suggested a test that might be used to determine a patient's interests (*Claire Conroy*, 1985). After recognizing that therapy can be ended for an incompetent patient "when it is clear that the particular patient would have refused the treatment under the circumstances involved," the court also introduced a "pure-objective test." This test, to be used when no trustworthy evidence, or no evidence at all, is available for determining what a person would have chosen, allows life-sustaining treatment to be either withheld or withdrawn when "the net burdens of the patient's life with the treatment . . . clearly and markedly outweigh the benefits that the patient derives from life." The court did not "authorize decision-making based on assessments of the personal worth or social utility of another's life, or the value of that life to another." The court also ruled that there are no differences between administering food and fluids and other medical therapies, nor any legal distinction between beginning therapy and ending therapy once it has begun (including the major concern of doctors—not starting a patient on a respirator versus taking a patient off the respirator at some later stage).

If we try to apply these recent court rulings to patients like Stephanie, we still remain in the grip of a hard problem. Stephanie has a very slight chance to survive. The court rulings do not address probabilities of successful treatment. Nor is it clear how to balance Stephanie's benefits and burdens in the context of her parents' strong desires to do everything for her. It is not even certain that a satisfactory account of interests can be given which focuses entirely on Stephanie to the exclusion of those committed to her welfare. The one clear implication of the courts' rulings, however, is that an effort must be made to determine her interests. To leave decisions on therapy entirely to Stephanie's parents is not enough.

2

March 22. Stephanie has many more lesions on her skin. These are probably the result of handling during surgery. Her nurse wonders whether they will heal—ever.

The Blackwell baby is being taken downstairs for a brain scan. Susan Markart tells me the baby seems to have a private on-off switch for reactions that operates independent of external stimuli. For example, she sleeps through a spinal tap (which ordinarily throws babies into a frenzy). She fights strenuously while being intubated—which is normal—but then in the middle of the session she suddenly relaxes for no observable reason. Also, Susan believes the baby is blind. There is some dispute over this among the nurses. It is very hard to tell. But the baby does not look at you or, indeed, at anything.

The nurse who is pregnant is in the level 2 wing. "You should have been here last Tuesday. I almost committed child abuse." What was the problem? "Oh, a chronic who went wild—for an hour and a half—when she didn't get her sedatives."

The temperature in Stephanie's room is kept between 90 and 94 degrees Fahrenheit. The heat is oppressive. It comes out of the room in a steady stream—a sauna for both staff and patient. Inside Stephanie lies naked on her side under a glass cover.

Many parents who visit the nursery seem tired and resigned, moving in slow motion. The mother of one baby who is hopeless—Brian O'Hara—looks hopeless herself as she sits by his bed holding his hand.

Michael Anthony is back from surgery, the stomach tube in place. Now he can be fed by inserting nourishment in a syringe, hooking the syringe to the gavage tube, and letting gravity take the nourishment into his stomach. Michael still has a catheter attached to him, his urine seeping down a plastic line. He is sweating a little. Mary Jane Kennedy: "He threw out his ventilator line—spit it out this morning. He's getting spoiled."

A nurse is bathing a baby who is on CPAP. He is being held up in a tub with a slight amount of water in it. The nurse is slowly washing him with a wash cloth. "He loves it—look, he's not even crying. You *love* it, don't you." The mother of this child calls as the nurse is toweling him off in his bed. "I'm not talking to her," the nurse calls out as she starts to suction the baby's nose and throat with a faulty suction device. "She called me just one hour ago." The other nurses start laughing. The nurse on the phone asks, "Shall I tell her that no one wants to talk to her?" *Yes*, everyone shouts. The nurse presses the phone receiver up against her chest. Then she resumes the conversation with the mother, her manner and voice strictly velvet. Afterwards she tells the other nurses that the mother had apologized for calling so much, but the day for her is so long and she can't stop thinking. The nurses will have none of it. "Let her come down and visit," one says without a trace of sympathy. "Suction her kid out awhile."

One of the interns is on her last day in the nursery. She is scheduled now for six weeks in the emergency room at the state hospital. She tells me that she is relieved at leaving the high-wire intensity of the nursery, and that she looks forward to a more relaxed existence at the emergency room (which puts into relief—like nothing else I've heard—the level of stress in neonatology).

Late at night I decide impulsively to stop by the nursery on the way home from the university. The nurses are engaged in horseplay as I enter, pushing each other and laughing. They say "Shh" as I walk by. I tell them, "Don't worry, I'm not working tonight."

There is a rich and wide range of human emotions present in the nursery. No surprise at this, for neonatology is a social practice with human beings acting in various guises toward each other. But the emotions change sharply at the boundaries of life-and-death situations. When, for example, Danielle Raymond almost died a few days ago, those working on her were loose and distant, employing their skills from some point outside pure emotions. They were intense, immensely competent, joking to relax, with no fear or sadness—more like performers with considerable talents than affected members of a human family. But when nurses handle babies on a routine basis they talk to the infants, express love, irritation, concern—the deep and full range of emotions that any good parent feels toward her children.

March 23. Stephanie's father is in the hall peering at his daughter through the window of her room, the back of his skin showing under his pulled up T-shirt.

Cindy Blackwell is being fed through a tube. In a scene merging medical technology with human affection, a nurse is gently rocking the baby in her lap as she holds aloft the syringe of nourishment. A sign for "Pizza Theatre" (a local pizza parlor and arcade for children) is on the side of the baby's bed.

Michael Anthony is asleep after (in Mary Jane Kennedy's words) "a long sleepless night." Kennedy is looking at Michael's monitor. It indicates the staccato irregularities of the baby's heartbeat. "Come on, Michael," she says. "Get out of it."

Danielle Raymond is on a ventilator, her body (at least to my unpracticed eyes) somewhat rigid. Any number of monitors are attached to her chest and abdomen. Her chart has check marks in every category of bodily activity—respiration, heart, temperature, etc.—as a sign for technicians to monitor these functions. In the bed next to her is a baby dressed in a pink cotton suit with a CPAP in her nose.

"You can't buy love" is being sung by the Beatles on the radio. A mother is wheeled in on her bed. She is attached to a mobile I.V. and is obviously exhausted. Her bed is placed next to the small crib where her baby—a few hours old—is lying. She holds her baby's foot with her left hand, caressing it while looking weakly at her child. This is the first time I feel like crying. A nurse comes over and tells her that her baby is over seven pounds, that her Apgar (a combined score on a number of indicators—color, pulse, reflex, muscle tone, and respiration) was a little low right after birth, and that they are just keeping the baby awhile for routine observation. The mother is then wheeled slowly out. If emotional settings are created by the different people in the nursery, than this mother has brought in a powerful set of parental emotions that are normally not present.

A message comes through on the telephone: Heather McCall has died in pediatrics. There is genuine shock in the nursery. Heather was a baby here two years ago. Originally just a premie (a premature baby), she developed extremely severe necrotizing enterocolitis, which required the removal of too much bowel. She suffered complications due to inadequate nourishment, and after two years of life in a hospital she is now dead. The word spreads quickly through the nursery and is met with dismay and sadness.

March 24. Stephanie is restless this afternoon. Her eyes are open, sometimes clouded with pain as she turns her face. It seems to me that consciousness is a kind of beacon that is blinding when it alights on you. Sometimes, as with Stephanie, this luminescence is present with an intensity felt by all. At other times, with other babies, the light is weak, turned inward. Why?

March 26. Michael Anthony was transferred today to a hospital in his hometown. He was running a fever earlier, so one nurse wondered whether he would actually leave. But the fever abated somewhat and off he went, respirator and all. Mary Jane Kennedy came in on her day off and accompanied him.

Brian is being rocked by a nurse when I enter his room. His eyes move up and to the left, seeming to focus on shapes somewhere in his field of vision. He is frowning, appears to be fearful of something. I imagine his brain as a flawed computer processing information in anomalous ways, constructing partial alternative realities of light and shadow. "Poor Brian" is the common referent around him.

Warren Carr went home on Saturday with his parents.

Stephanie is, once again, "doing as well as can be expected." She has multiple blisters on her skin. She is lying on her side, her two hands raised in a supplicating position above and near her face. Vaseline gauzes are wrapped loosely on her forearm and lower legs and ankles. Her rib cage moves in and out as she breathes. There is a single line now in her abdomen to supply her with all her worldly needs. She is an earthling with a space cord controlling her drift, connected to the mother ship.

3

The quality and future of Stephanie's life are problems for everyone who comes into contact with her. No one knows how to weigh her interests in deciding whether to continue or stop her therapy. Nor is it clear how the therapy can be stopped without violating accepted rules of medical care. She is alive. Her neurological functions are intact. She is a human being with all of the rights to life accorded to other human beings in Western societies. Yet her pain and bleak prospects might lead a rational adult to say, "Enough"—and choose death. Stephanie cannot make this choice, nor affirm its opposite— life—as a choice. Whoever decides for her will have to make very fine decisions on benefits versus burdens, and perhaps even examine quality-of-life conditions in general, for Stephanie can have no thoughts on whether her particular life is worth living.

Some would say that all life is worth living. The Right to Life Foundation is founded precisely on the proposition that the value of life is unconditional, not to be ended by intentional action no matter what its quality. But there are physical extremes that make one wonder. Terminal pain can be so intense as to make death merciful. And some forms of human life will make anyone question whether the life represented is worth maintaining no matter what. A traditional philosophy would say that nature or God must resolve such matters. But the skills of neonatologists have taken us far beyond natural beginnings and endings. The issue in Stephanie's case is how much support should be given to a child whom nature would have claimed some time ago in the absence of modern medicine.

Society does not permit individuals to make all decisions on medical therapy. Where the good to the community outweighs the risks of therapy, individuals are sometimes coerced into accepting medical treatment. Measles vaccine, for example, provides a small but real risk to all who are innoculated. If children do not get vaccinated, however, they are not permitted to attend school in many states. In this type of case, even rational individuals are not allowed to decide without costs whether to accept the medical risks of innoculation. When communicable disease is not at issue, the state will mandate treatment if rational competence is not demonstrated. In these areas the society regulates individual choice for the good of the individual. If the individual is competent, able to decide for himself, and if the state is not responsible in some special way for his well-being, the choices on therapy may be free of regulation. The law, on those conditions, recognizes the individual's right to weigh life against its qualities.

How the balance is set, however, may be used as an indication of competence. The individual in New York who decided not to have his feet partially amputated as treatment for frostbite because God would care for him was, in large part because of his decision, judged incompetent. A competent decision must be reasonable, or in accord with a rough set of beliefs about rational trade-offs of life and its qualities (intact feet, presumably, not considered so strong a quality as to risk death for). Not all idiosyncratic beliefs on therapy are regulated by the state. Jehovah's Witnesses, for example, can still refuse blood transfusions on religious grounds. But when decisions are made on behalf of others, the limits on choice are more severely drawn (demonstrated whenever parents try—unsuccessfully—to deny transfusions for their children on religious grounds). Like a fiduciary relationship, the decisions on therapy for another seem bound by conservative norms, and what is most worth conserving in all such decisions is life itself.

What are reasonable beliefs on the conditions for continuing life? One, accepted by all physicians interviewed, is that errors toward life are better than errors against life. If a child has any chance to survive intact this chance must be played out. Such a belief provides an incentive for early aggressive treatment, when diagnostic uncertainty is greatest. But the early stages of Stephanie's condition have passed. Her doctors are now approaching a reasonable certainty that she will not survive. One of the ironies of Stephanie's disease is that what is normally the main condition for a reasonable life accepted by both staff and parents is present in her life. Her brain, as far as anyone knows, is not damaged in any way.

Other quality-of-life considerations do not bear on Stephanie's condition. After an intact brain, the most frequently mentioned quality is mobility, in the larger sense of independence—from machines and others. The thought of spending one's entire life shackled to a ventilator or on I.V. is repulsive to most physicians. Then there is longevity, which seems always mediated by other conditions. A short life, to most, is better than no life. But if this brief existence is one of immobility and pain, then there is an even stronger reason to say that treatment makes no sense. Pain itself, however, is not so important. Like neurological deficits, it is characterized by gradations that make decisions of therapy very fine indeed. But, unlike neurological problems, pain can be alleviated by modern medicine.

From an interview with Bonnie Sorenson, an intern in the nursery. Sorenson is a competent, no-nonsense woman in her twenties. She is without ~~affections~~. affectations.

Sorenson: Pain, does pain count? From a day-to-day basis, does pain count in the unit? When we're dealing with children, it doesn't count at all because we inflict pain. That's something that I, as an intern, have to deal with. It's very difficult for me to deal with. On a day-to-day basis, day after day after day, hour after hour, I'm doing painful procedures on these children routinely, and you don't even think about it after a while. I mean you think about it every time, but it doesn't in any way make you reconsider whether the tests need to be done if you feel medically they need to be done. It doesn't enter into the equation. Does pain count in terms of deciding whether a child's life should be prolonged? Physical pain, emotional pain, what kind of pain are we talking about?

Frohock: Start with physical pain.

Sorenson: Does it count? Yes, but I can't really put it in tangible terms in my mind, in terms of thinking of a specific medical condition that would be so overwhelmingly painful for a protracted period of time and would not be able to be relieved . . .

Frohock: How about Stephanie? What can she anticipate in the way of pain?

Sorenson: I don't think Stephanie can anticipate much in the way of longevity, period. I think Stephanie right now is experiencing a lot of pain. Pain is very interesting—because does pain involve having higher cerebral functions than children at this age have? What is pain in these kids? What I've been told for the few children who do survive the disease Stephanie has, the lesions clear. So there isn't a course of unremitting pain to look forward to. And many of the physical handicaps that we deal with also aren't a matter of day-in and day-out pain. It's just a matter of being debilitated—of lessening what you can do in a very practical sense. I'm not trying to be evasive. I don't know if I can give an answer because I have a difficult time just answering in the abstract. I really can't think of a tangible condition where that is an overwhelming factor.

Frohock: Let me go to another factor. Morphology—human form. Does that count? What about children who will grow up to be severely disfigured?

Sorenson: I don't think disturbing the aesthetics of other people should count, no.

The list of quality-of-life conditions, however, is misleading unless qualified and extended with three observations. First, neurological functions are not merely the first on an ordinal listing of quality-of-life conditions. They dwarf all other conditions in cardinal magnitude. The brain is far and away the most important organ of life for all respondents. Second, that physicians mention secondary conditions like mobility does not mean that they act on such beliefs toward their patients. The overwhelming bias of physicians—by training and instruction—is toward preserving life. As Susan Markart put it: "I will go ahead and resuscitate because my training is to take care of those babies. I'm a pediatrician and that's what I do. I save lives." Also, the physicians do not make decisions on therapy alone. The parents contribute their views. Third, the question of how to reduce or discontinue therapy constrains the weighing of life against its qualities. This question is particularly important in the case of Stephanie, for there is not that much therapy to discontinue in her case.

There is another thought that instructs us on the role of quality-of-life considerations in therapy decisions. The thought begins with a recognition of three different types of decisions. One type is formed from expert knowledge. If elevators malfunction on a college campus, maintenance people are called in. They repair the elevators according to the laws of Newtonian mechanics and for a level of performance set by safety standards. Elevator repair may not be an axiomatic science, but decisions within the field are governed by precise standards that allow the recognition of experts. The second type of decision is conditioned by rights. If two claimants appear before a judge in a dispute over access to one or the other's property, the judge will try to determine the rights of each individual. The legal decision will follow a recognition (and possible adjustment) of property rights and rights of liberty.

The use of quality-of-life considerations in therapy does not seem to fit either of these types of decisions. Neither precise standards nor rights is a helpful resource for therapy decisions in hard cases. The decisive terms that might permit expert decisions—*quality*, perhaps *arete* (excellence)—are discussed at length by the Sophists of ancient Greece (and by Robert Persig in his marvelous book, *Zen and the Art of Motorcycle Maintenance*). But the conclusions of that discussion have been lost or abandoned in medical therapy. Today there is legitimate dispute over what constitutes quality in human life. There *is* a convergence of beliefs among doctors and parents that neurological functions are the most important items to have intact (thus continuing the emphasis in classical philosophy on *nous*—intellect or thinking as the locus for the person). But the convergence is merely an agreement among certain participants in the neonatal nursery. There is no independent principle that provides an exact balance between life and quality of life, no standard of the sort that we use to set safety minimums for elevator mainte-nance. Nor do the rights of concerned parties seem important in therapy decisions. To say that infants have a right to life sets the thresholds of no-code decisions at very high levels. But acknowl-edging that a baby like Stephanie has a right to life does not tell us when treatment is no longer humane or even intelligible. Therapy decisions in the difficult, gray area of choice seem to resemble a third type of decision, represented by decisions that set utility rates or establish obligations to future generations. Instead of an exact prin-ciple or a set of rights, there is a requirement: find and state general constraints within which a consensus can be forged on how to proceed.

It is not even certain that an agreement on quality could empty out the hard cases in therapy. They may always be with us as hard cases. Imagine a map of goods that represent a social consensus on quality. In Homeric societies these goods would include success in both war and peace. Health in a Homeric society would be an enabling good, one that allows individuals to secure life's qualities. But it does not follow that the grid connecting enabling goods to the map of qualities could be plotted with precision. Various infirmities, for example epilepsy, might permit success, and other infirmities, for example pain, might actually connect dramatically to some of the quality goods. It might still be impossible to say with certainty what the connections are between states of health and life's qualities even when society agrees on what these qualities are.

The *Storar* ruling tells us that representatives do not have full discretionary authority to define the interests of those they repre-sent. The merits of a case, or some more general statement on interests, must guide decisions. But *quality*, the term that might be helpful in providing some guidance, has no definition that all can accept. And it is not even clear that a consensus on quality would elminate hard cases. So we are left with an interesting problem. We are not clones of one another, and so no one is a perfect surrogate for anyone else. But because of our differences we must find a way to agree on some non-Newtonian constraints on therapy decisions, or accept the unsettling fact that therapy is purely a discretionary practice.

From an interview with Joe Ritiglia.

Frohock: Most of the cases we've talked about in the last few minutes involve neurological deficiencies—deficits I think is the phrase that's used. We have a case now of a baby with a skin disorder, presumably intact neurologically.

Ritiglia: I think that's one of the stickiest kinds of issues. So much of it is subjective. All right, that's a baby who we're assuming is intact neurologically. Her problem is that she has a skin disorder where she forms blisters. The skin sloughs off and leaves a lot of open, draining wounds essentially, with tremendous fluid losses. Now the nature of her specific illness is such that things are not going to result in scarring. So we're not even dealing with a potential for a disfigured baby afterwards. But it subjectively appears very uncomfortable. The quality of life now is horrendous. The baby has no human contact; is intermittently seen by caretakers with gloves and masks, gowns; is on a bed in a warm room; has none of the things which go into the development of a normal baby. That in and of itself may cause some developmental problems. Nobody knows and it's not hard and fast. Maybe it's a thing that can be overcome, so I wouldn't really put a loss on it. But it's something to tuck away in the back of the mind.

Medically, the baby is very difficult to manage because of all the fluid loss, protein loss. The baby's not eating. Remember it had that congenital problem with the intestines and needed surgery early on. But somehow it seems that you should be able to—maybe, maybe not—but in the sort of egocentric view of the physician, there should be something that can be done in a kid like this medically. You should be able to figure it out somehow—how to manage the fluids, how to provide the nutrition. That's what's been going on. Every day go through it all over again. Figure out the nutrition. Try something new. Try a different kind of food. Intravenous feedings are being continued. Check the blood work. You do everything that needs to be done. So that you've got it. But what you've got in the meantime is a baby who has simultaneously the potential for survival with a horrendous quality of life subjectively at this point in time.

Now we can't ask this baby "Are you in pain?" "Is this enough?" Do you say enough is enough? Can we ask that of the mother? At what point does the mother say enough is enough? What if a mother just has a low tolerance of pain? She says "I can't stand to see my kid suffer." That happens sometimes. They just overreact. A baby who's moderately ill but clearly has an excellent chance for survival with a normal outcome, mothers will totally lose it when they get blood work drawn or routine I.V.'s or something which you know is going to leave no scars. So we can't totally leave it to the mother or the parents to say, "Look, enough is enough." Because what are their limits? You don't know their limits, so you've got to have some interaction yourself.

I think in a kid like this, the way I would do it would be to judge the potential for medical management. Let's just suppose that I had been involved with Stephanie and I realized I had been doing absolutely everything that I could do. That I tried everything that I could try and we were still slipping. The course just seemed inexorably headed towards death even with everything I could do. Now that's something that you have to judge from the perspective of the ongoing management of the baby. There's not a miracle cure that's going to come up in the next week. That's not going to happen. So I think if you've experienced that and you say look, every day it slowly gets a little bit worse. It's not two steps forward and one step back. It's two steps back and one step forward. Then I think I'd say enough is enough.

Again, this just becomes intensely difficult for the family to deal with. And, again, this situation, this is a baby with parents who've had a previous child with it. And then you have to decide—which is probably what has happened. They have decided that they would continue to make this baby as comfortable as possible, to do what we can. But should a catastrophe occur, we don't intervene to make further problems. It may be that in another couple of weeks of the same thing happening, they're going to say enough is enough. And if we stopped giving our I.V.'s, or gave I.V. fluids and oxygen and pain medication but not nutrition, or just gave her maintenance fluids and didn't replace the losses that she's having through her skin, that instead of us being able to keep her alive for another month, maybe it would last for a few days or a week. That may be a transition that takes place.

Frohock: And if the parents at the beginning had said, "Don't treat," what would the attending physician have done right at the beginning?

Ritiglia: That's a good question. I think if, as the physician, you think that there's a potential for survival with a reasonable quality of life ultimately, you've got to try to convince them that it's worth trying. This is something that does come up—"I don't want my baby to be subjected to anything." Then you've got to decide how off the wall are the parents? And you've got to have an understanding of the process of the disease, which unfortunately I don't have in Stephanie's. Not many people do. But I think I would as rapidly as possible accumulate that knowledge by dealing with the appropriate consultants. And then if the parents say, "I don't want anything done to this baby," and you know that if you do something this baby has a reasonable chance for a good survival, then you've got to decide about legal intervention. I hope that would never happen to me because I think that would be just so damaging to the family. But it's done. What that would mean would be taking the baby from the custody of the family and putting it in the custody of the courts—the judge then saying "Doctor, do what you should do." I don't think that's the end of the world. I would have a tremendously hard time, emotionally, doing that. In a kid with chemotherapy whom that happened to, the family just left the child. They've maintained contact, begrudgingly. But the bond—it still exists between the family and the child. They just think that the wrong thing is being done and they suffer with it.

From an interview with Randy Hunter.

Hunter: One of the difficulties I have with this, and with children with deformities and all that kind of thing, is any group or any person making a statement for a child. Saying, "Well, if the kid can't walk or if he can't talk or if he can't hear, I know if I couldn't see, I wouldn't want to live. So I know this kid's okay but blind, but I don't think we ought to treat him because who wants to be raised blind all their life." Well, you can go out and get testimonies from a lot of blind folks who say they'd rather be alive and blind than dead. They'd rather get a chance to live than not live. On the other hand, a child that is going to go through fifteen or twenty operations in the first three years of life, whose mental function will never be above—will never be able to read, may be able to speak a few words—how can you say whether that kid's emotional input and output is enough to have the kid at one point say "Well, I'm glad I'm alive.

From an interview with Joe Ritiglia.

Frohock: Let me ask you a question about quality of life. If you had a kind of laundry list on the conditions you think are necessary to have a reaonable life, what would head your list and what would you include on it?

Ritiglia: See, the more I learn, the more limited the list becomes. I think number one would have to be an ability to have relationships with other human beings. In my mind, to love or receive love, to have sort of a role in a group, be it a family or some place, I think is the key. Whether you can hold a job, I don't know. I'd like to see that done without a lot of physical suffering. I'd like to see the potential for some development and that just means ending up in a different place from where you started. It doesn't necessarily mean an IQ of 130. Again, the anecdotes come back. My sister-in-law had a child with Down's syndrome when she was twenty-two and there's a kid with—who knows what's going to happen. And the first couple of years he was an infant and that's easy. But he didn't walk until late and still doesn't really talk well. I think his quality of life is excellent. It's going to be tough on him as he gets older and he'll know it and it's not easy on the family. But he's loved and he loves his family. . . .

Even more extreme, I took care of a child who's ten years old with severe, severe cerebral palsy. I mean the worst muscle wasting, stiff, contractures like a pretzel, whose family just carried her around; who lived at home the whole time and they talk about her and everybody took turns feeding her. She had a gastronomy tube. She didn't really eat but she was alive. She was more a repository for emotion than one who provides it. But she served a role in that family. She really brought the family together. When this kid was hospitalized, her brother, who was in the service, took a leave to come and see her. I don't understand that. Is that quality of life? Whose quality of life?

Frohock: Would you then look at the quality of the family in determining the quality of life for an individual?

Ritiglia: I can't go that far in that direction either. Because how do you put a qualitative analysis on a family? I don't think I can really do that. It's like somebody could give a brilliant speech in Greek and I would have no idea whether it was brilliant or not. People just love in different languages and in different ways and I can't say what's right and wrong. I think you'd have to lead it on an individual basis. It's a very difficult question to answer. I had a baby with terrible birth asphyxia who was on a respirator for days and finally came off and really is going to have troubles indefinitely. The parents were actively involved and really cared. They wanted this kid no matter what. Does this kid have the chance for a quality of life? I don't know, but I would never think of withdrawing support from him. The family unit existed. I don't know whether this is right or not. You read about people who try to set guidelines, some objectivity to it, something that can be applied to people sort of across the board. I've just not been able to find that in my own experience.

The interviews show that decisions to continue, reduce, or stop therapy once it has begun are not neat exercises of life weighed against its conditions. Such decisions are the outcomes of protracted negotiations between physicians and parents where a variety of measures, balances, and compromises are considered. In most cases the surrogate of the child is the physician-parent group. The interests of the child that are typically expressed by this group are usually some amalgam of medical need and parental wishes emerging from discussion within the group.

The variables of these discussions are identifiable, even though their values differ among cases. One is neurology—whether and how the brain of the child is working. Another is the capacity of the child to live in some way free of the medical technology that continues her life. These two variables are interpreted by the attitude of parents—how, in general, they respond to and support the child. Stated roughly, the treatment thresholds of neural capacity and mobility are set by the willingness of the parents to push for therapy and accept their children.

From an interview with Randy Hunter.

Frohock: Suppose I set up two poles—those who believe in life no matter what and those who are influenced in therapy by quality-of-life considerations. The number 10 is life-no-matter-what, and 1 stands for a variety of quality-of-life conditions. Where are most doctors on this continuum?

Hunter: How they behave would range 5 to 8, maybe 6 to 8. Well, 5 to 8.

Frohock: Where would you place yourself?

Hunter: Six, maybe 7. I mean just by—see, by the time you get to either end, I think you have fools, not physicians. I think somebody that's a 9 or a 10 or a 1 or a 2 is ignorant of the human condition and those people disgust me.

March 27. Stephanie is to be baptized today. Fearing the worst, I ask why. Because her parents (who are here at the moment) are trying to extend their insurance coverage through the state and need either a birth certificate or a baptismal certificate to do it. They are protecting themselves with the baptismal certificate. So what is (presumably) a natural inclination of the parents to have a priest come in is fortified by pragmatic considerations. The priest, by the way, has to use water that is both holy and sterile in giving the sacrament—a rare convergence of secular and spiritual purity. Stephanie is on her side resting right now, her white bed covering still fluttering lightly in the breeze that is constantly coming up to hold the bed spheres level. When the priest comes in, he is handed a white hospital gown and mask to place over her vestments. Inside her room he sprinkles water on Stephanie, his lips moving in prayers that cannot be heard through the glass window. He is heavy and solemn in his bearing. The entire ritual takes less than three minutes. Afterwards Stephanie's mother seems agitated. She comes over and tells a nurse that her son (with her in the nursery) has a temperature of 102. They (father, mother, son) are advised to leave for the Ronald McDonald house (where they are staying). Stephanie has slept through everything.

Do babies get the flu from ill visitors? Yes, I am told, but no one knows it. If their condition drops, if they are infected, the doctors simply give them antibiotics.

Doctors have special interests in certain diseases. Susan Markart's is metabolic diseases, a subject on which she is currently holding forth in the hall. Doctors seem to bond with disorders the way nurses bond with babies.

Julia Allen, the famous baby filled accidentally with intralipid, is now getting oxygen from only a hood. She weighed only 560 grams five months ago and needed substantial ventilator support. Now she is at 2780 grams and successfully weaned from the ventilator. In spite of the improvement, children like Julia are difficult. They take a good hour to feed, are irritable, subject to frequent infections. They have chronic lung problems. "Parents have to be saints to care for them," a nurse observes. "They are good candidates for child abuse." As adults they tend to suffer from emphysema. From childhood forward there are frequent returns to a hospital for respiratory therapy. It is a hard life.

The nurse caring for Stephanie tells me that "her thighs are gone"—meaning scraped away in lesions. She is also losing skin on her back and under her arms due to (necessary) increased handling. The doctors are worried more now about infections.

It is easy to think, looking at Stephanie, that her life is not beneficial to her. She knows little else but pain. No one expects her to live much longer. Wouldn't it be humane to put an end to her suffering rather than let her linger on before dying of infection? Only three options are open. One is to continue to treat her aggressively in order to prolong her life as long as possible. A second is to cut back on therapy to some modest point, or to decide not to begin certain therapies if a need arises later. The third is to intervene and end her suffering by ending her life.

Many of the distinctions between passive and active euthanasia do not bear on Stephanie's case. The *intention* to do harm, or to kill, seems not very helpful in most cases where euthanasia is considered. If a child is (a) injected with lethal potassium, or (b) taken away from a needed antibiotic or respirator, the intention in both cases is to hasten the death of the child. There is one important difference between the two acts. Active intervention with lethal substances removes all possibility for the patient to continue living. Failing to administer an antibiotic or turning off a respirator still permits the patient to live (as was discovered in the Karen Ann Quinlan case). Passive euthanasia in this way is more tolerant of error. No one can be absolutely sure that Stephanie won't yet survive her ordeal. And so no one is about to administer a lethal injection.

But even if one were certain about outcomes, there still might be hesitation in allowing active euthanasia. Several doctors believe that the practice would erode respect for life itself. Respect for life is one of the deep values of medicine. Why, for example, do we assume that, in most circumstances, individuals ought to consent to therapy? Because we believe that individuals have dignity and intrinsic worth, are to be treated as ends and not means, and have inalienable rights, among which are life and liberty. Absent these beliefs and these are no important reasons to allow individuals to control their own lives as autonomous agents. This high standing of the individual person in western social practices makes the interest of the patient paramount in medicine and creates dilemmas when patients cannot fulfill autonomy (as comatose patients and infant children cannot). It is precisely the values assigned to individuals that compel respect for life itself. The high standing of life is normally accepted as more important than the humanitarian desire to end suffering through active enthanasia.

The arguments for some form of euthanasia are more persuasive when the treatment itself is useless or damaging, or where the patient is beyond salvation in any intact form. Treatment can be painful but justified because of its ultimately beneficial effects. But treatment that is painful with no benefits, or that itself causes harm, or that merely prolongs the suffering of patients, or that is aiming to maintain a patient with inadequate neurological functions, may not make sense on any rational or moral test. Withdrawing such therapy may be justified by the same respect for life that informs resistance to euthanasia. Each decision on withdrawing support must be endorsed by both doctors and parents, making euthanasia in any of its forms subordinate to often complicated consent formulas. As a general rule, however, to die with dignity seems a corollary value to individual worth.

The euthanasia decisions in the nursery are always passive. The staff will withhold certain therapies once they have decided (along with the parents) that the therapies are no longer in the interests of the patient. No one believes that all levels of life are worth living no matter what. But the uncertainty over what levels *are* worth living (as well as uncertainty over prognosis) makes these decisions cautious and incremental.

One wonders if the right questions are asked in settling on a patient's interests when deciding on life-maintaining therapies. Instead of asking whether an individual's life is of benefit to the individual, we might ask—while maintaining the recognized values of dignity and self-worth—is a person's life meaningful in some human context? Does Stephanie's (or anyone's) existence make sense only in terms of her effect on others? And does such a view of individuals reframe the issues of euthanasia in both its passive and active forms?

I encounter Mary Jane Kennedy in the hall. "Don't talk to me," she says. Why, I ask. "Michael just arrested. Twice this morning." Is he okay now? "He's alive." Kennedy is obviously overwrought. She found out about the arrests in the worst possible way. A cardiologist dropped by the nursery this morning and casually remarked that Michael Anthony had almost died earlier in the day. Kennedy got the rest of the story by calling the hospital to which the child had been moved. She tells me that Michael's arrests are caused by the move itself to a different hospital. "He doesn't know where he is. Someone is caring for him whom he doesn't know."

Later I hear this account discussed by some doctors. They say that a move will frequently upset the electrolyte balance of a child, and this, not the sense of loss, was the more likely source of Michael's arrests. Still, it is an interesting possibility. Michael Anthony may know Mary Jane Kennedy. And he may know that she loves him. So, although he is severely brain-damaged and in a disastrous physical condition, he may interact with his environment. On this hypothesis, he exists in a world, and in this world he receives affection and gives affection in his recognition of Kennedy and his favored treatment of her in allowing only her to treat him. He may now die in a sort of shock and grief at losing this world. He is, on this account of things, a child whose life has meaning in the context of human lives that he affects in important ways.

6
Human Identity

1

What makes us human is a puzzle that has been addressed since the beginnings of recorded thought. Perhaps to be a thinking, reflective creature is to be able to ask what one is. But if efforts at self-definition are part of what is meant by the human condition, it is by that measure discouraging that the answers we provide are so different from one another. Our deepest, most important inquiry—defining ourselves—has yielded only disagreement.

The magnitude of the disagreement can be seen in current discussions over humanness. One important (and provocative) set of human criteria has been proposed by Joseph Fletcher, in his 1972 article "Indicators of Humanhood" (See Bibliography, section 5). Fletcher suggests a "profile of man" in fifteen positive and five negative propositions. The positive items are all extensions of neocortical functions, including such features as minimal intelligence, self-awareness, self-control, a sense of time, a sense of futurity, a sense of the past, the capability to relate to others, and so on. The negative items are curious indeed, stating such propositions as that man is not essentially parental, sexual, a bundle of rights, a worshiper. The tests are clearly biased toward Fletcher's own model of humanness. "Curiosity," for example, is number 11 on the list, a "concern for others" number 8—all laudable traits, but unfortunate news for the dull and self-centered individual who labors under the (apparent) illusion that he is a human being. One might also quarrel with the negative view of either (or both) sexual or worshiper tests—or, for that matter, with any of the tests Fletcher advances. But the specific items are less important than the core idea Fletcher has seized. Though he inexplicably lists neocortical function as a criterion, it is best seen as the core proposition in the set of features: that to be human is to be a thinking, reflective creature.

The life of the mind has been central to western understanding of humanness in centuries of law and morality. Both Plato and Aristotle defined our humanness in terms of rational thought, that capacity for reflection that they believed (and we believe) marks us off from other animals. Legal determinations of diminished personhood always turn on reduced mental capacity. A man who loses his arms, his legs, any part of his body, is not in law considered less of a person as a consequence of the loss. But neurological deficits may render him legally impaired, his judgments transferable to a guardian who can decide for him.

The problem of using rational thought as an indicator of humanness is its scalar quality. We can be more or less thoughtful. Are we more or less human as a result? Here the terrain is difficult and (rightly) controversial. Brain-damaged adults may not have full legal status as persons. They may even become wards of others. But we do not view them as less than human. Then there is the matter of children. Since the brain is an organ that, like all forms of life, develops according to biological laws, consciousness—of self, of others—emerges over time. Do we become humans only as our brains develop their full capacities? And what of those humans whose brains never develop to a reasonable capacity? If the world were organized into static units of life, then scale would not be the moral problem it is. But the brain is developmental, with the possibility of error and failure encoded into the developmental patterns. Do the errors and failures diminish humanness?

These questions become even more difficult as we explore what follows from defining humans in terms of the cerebral cortex. The story that begins with rational thought as the test of humanness ends today with the assignment of rights to individuals on the basis of their neocortical functions. The key right is the right to life. But here are the seeds of a problem. If a certain level of neurological activity is a qualification for being human, then those forms of life which do not realize the level may forfeit the right to life accorded to humans routinely. Among these forms are children, brain-damaged adults, neurologically defective persons of any age.

One can of course accept what most regard as unacceptable—that human beings who do not meet certain neurological thresholds are really not human. But such an acceptance offends both law and morality. The point of self-definition is not to exclude member of the human community but to recognize a language that extends to those who are morally and legally accepted as human. One way to correct the error of exclusion (leaving out those whom we want to include) is to accept an error of inclusion: set the level of neurologi-cal activity so low as to cover a wide range of brain deficiency, including the absence of a cerebral cortex (which is Warren Carr's problem). The error here, if it can be called that, is that a level of neurological activity set low enough to include Warren Carr will also include many higher-vertebrate animals—apes, chimpanzees, gorillas, dogs, cats. But perhaps this inclusion is not an error. The error may be in assuming that the human species is special, separate from all other forms of life. An inclusive definition of humanness at least recognizes the continuity of life. It tells us that we are part of an animal world that may have claims to the respect for life currently reserved to the human species almost exclusively.

The rules of treatment in the nursery are not affected by defini-tions of humanness. Every baby in the nursery is treated, even those without a brain. No thought is ever expressed on whether a baby is human. All are assumed to be human by virtue of being born of human parents. The simplicity of the assumption appeals. Human-ness is not assigned to the individual baby but to the family of the baby. If pressed, the staff will tend to define humanness in terms of physical tests, like chromosomal counts and arrangements. These physical tests do, at some level, demarcate humans from nonhuman forms of life. The individual born of such physical human speci-mens, then, need not meet any additional tests, say for neurological activity. He is a member of a human community by virtue of his progenitor.

The problem with all such minimal physical tests for humanness is that they do not capture what it is to be a human being. Some mental or spiritual activity seems essential to human life (leading some philosophers to distinguish "human being" from "human person"). It is not clear, however, what this activity is that all higher vertebrates share, nor how mental or spiritual activities can be defined.

March 29. I was in the nursery for two hours this morning. Slow. Of course I can't wish crises on the staff just for the sake of my own research.

Conversations with Mary Jane Kennedy. "Michael Anthony's mother called me on Tuesday night to ask how *I* was. I was mor-tified. I was determined not to break down in front of her on the telephone." Kennedy tells me that she broke up with her fiancé last month and only Michael Anthony kept her going. It is clear even to me (I am not a psychologist) that Kennedy is deeply, perhaps dangerously, involved with Michael Anthony. I hope she knows what is going on with her emotions. Michael Anthony is now reported to be stable.

Brian O'Hara's CAT scan came back this morning showing very little brain growth, practically no cerebrum. He is whining softly at this moment, sounding like a cat on a ventilator. Eyes not seeing anything delineated in the world. Now one eye closes. He appears thoughtful without thought. Opposite his bed is one where Deborah sleeps, a child of the leading cardiologist in the hospital. Kennedy calls her "the best dressed baby on the floor."

One baby in the level 1 wing is the child of a diabetic mother. These babies are quite large. They get excessive insulin during gestation. Then their blood sugar plummets after birth. They must be weaned off their sugar dependence like a drug addict is slowly taken off heroin. The doctors send a sugar solution into their bloodstream and then slowly reduce the sugar content until their systems are back to normal. If the babies survive these early problems they do fine. They have no greater chance for diabetes than do individuals without diabetic parents.

So many babies in the nursery are peppered with marks on their skin where needles have been inserted to draw blood or provide medicine and nourishment. It is a mistake to underestimate the pain and discomfort that babies suffer here in the unit.

An intern is about to draw blood from a baby. "Ready to donate?" he murmurs as he clips a needle to a glass vial. "If you pee on me you're in trouble," he tells the baby as he inserts the needle under her skin.

Stephanie now has bandages around her ribs and under her arms as well as those still around her forehead and ankles. She is a beautiful baby—in spite of all this or because of it? I swear her spirit can be felt whenever one comes near her. Michael Anthony's spirit is brooding, underground. Though it has the power to control Mary Jane Kennedy.

March 30. Danielle Raymond looks like a guppy, her mouth opening and shutting on the ventilator tube. An "I survived Darien Lake" button is pinned to her bed sheets.

Cindy Blackwell is deep in a sleep that may be close to coma, though she ascends from these depths very quickly when disturbed. The nurses have hand-printed a sign that hangs from her crib: "If you wake me, you have to do whatever it takes to get me back to sleep." Her crib is now cluttered with toys. Two Fisher-Price boats are on the bed, a mobile of a horses-only merry-go-round hangs from a sheet placed over the front part of the crib. A nurse tells me that most of the toys are provided by the nursery. I can't understand why.

Michael Jackson's "Thriller" is on Y-94, a local radio station specializing in popular music. Vincent Price's voice competes with the staff conversations as he describes the possibilities of terror and the unknown.

March 31. Stephanie's bandages are being changed. She gets morphine now each time they handle her. She is twisted with pain. There is an ugly gash behind her left thigh. She is truly a burn victim day after day after day.

Julia Allen is turning blue, gasping for breath. Her mouth is opening and closing. A nurse is pounding on her chest and back. After about ten minutes of pounding she is breathing more normally through the freshly cleared tracheal tubes. Another nurse approaches holding a pad and pen. "It's about time I wrote notes on Julia." She leans over one inch from the baby's face. "I have to write notes on you." Pause. "You don't care, do you?"

Mary Jane Kennedy answers the red phone. She listens. "What?" Several nurses gather near her. She hangs up. "It's a thirty-seven-weeker that looks like a thirty-three-weeker. The mother is fifteen." Another nurse shakes her head. Kennedy nods. "I know. Fifteen. I wasn't even hardly kissing when I was fifteen."

It is a slow Saturday afternoon, sunny and warm outdoors though with snow still on the ground. The nurses open one of the windows in room A. Things are starting to pick up in the nursery. The nurses complain about incomings, but they thrive on the excitement. If they suffer burnout, it is because of the emotional attachments they form with the babies, not because of the pace. The doctors, more distant from the babies emotionally, do not suffer as much from this type of stress.

Brian was moved to a regional hospital yesterday to be nearer his parents. A healthy baby—a "pit-stop" baby (here only briefly to be checked)—is in the crib he has vacated. The new baby is crying lustily. The nurses say he is used to being nursed and he is hungry. Unfortunately they have been instructed not to feed him for two more hours so that his intestinal tract can be examined. Everyone is jumpy from his crying, but it is the jumpiness that is found around normal babies who are expressing strong and normal needs.

April 2. Stephanie is not doing well. She sleeps at the moment unattended, bandages soaked in vaseline covering her arms, legs, abdomen. The parts of her skin that are uncovered are swabbed with amnion. Her face is burrowed up against her right arm, which is folded just under her nose. Two tubes extend from her body. One is a thick yellow line going directly into her abdomen. It is for feeding. The other is a thin white line penetrating an area of her skin just above her breastbone. This second line is used for fluids and medication. Many lesions and red spots on her exposed skin make her look like she has an early case of chicken pox. A patch of blue paper—an open package of diapers—is gently blowing in the hot air coming off of Stephanie's bed. There is no other movement in the room.

Stephanie's problems keep multiplying. Her protein level is one-third what it should be and the doctors have been unable to raise it. Fluids are being pumped into her as rapidly as possible. But, since protein helps keep fluid in the body (and is itself lost through open wounds), the fluid pumped into her is oozing out through her skin and even into her skin. The loss of fluid through her many lesions is simply depleting the protein more rapidly that it can be replaced. Yesterday the burn service at the hospital came up with a new treatment for Stephanie. This afternoon they will begin applying a semisynthetic substance called biobrane. In burn patients the substance works as a skin substitute that promotes healing while reducing body fluid loss and decreasing the incidence of additional skin abrasions. Everyone hopes that the new treatment will help. A consensus is growing, however, that Stephanie is slipping away. Earlier today her parents, nurses, and physicians had a discussion. Everyone agreed that full treatment should be continued for Stephanie for every condition that is correctable. If she gets an infection, she is to be given antibiotics. Her electrolytes are to be kept in balance. Fluid loss is to be replaced. She is to be given bicarbonates for acidosis. Her hyperalimentation (including intralipid) is to continue. She is to be kept on the Clinitron bed. The oxygen face mask is to be used continuously. She will be manually stimulated for apnea. Her skin will continue to be treated. She will get morphine for pain and narcan to counter the effects of too much morphine. But the parents and staff have agreed that Stephanie is not to be treated if her condition dramatically worsens. If, for example, she has a major decompensation and her heart stops, no one will make an effort to bring her back from that type of deterioration. There will be no CPR (cardiopulmonary rescussitation) and no use of vasoactives (neither epinephrine to stimulate the heart or dopamine to increase blood pressure). Nor will she be bagged or put on a ventilator. The medical opinion is that it would be impossible to get her back if she suffers a major systemic failure.

Stephanie is obviously losing her battle.

2

An incident occurred last year at the hospital that is still discussed by the staff. At an outlying hospital a baby was born suffering from respiratory distress and some other problems that the attending obstetrician could not handle. The baby was transported to the neonatology nursery at Northeastern General. There the baby's condition worsened. At one point the attending physician judged the baby to be beyond salvation. He advised the parents to accept a no-code (do not resuscitate) instruction on therapy. After an agonizing period of reflection and discussion, the parents agreed. But the hospital administration, fearful at the time of legal action by the Reagan administration, ordered that full treatment of the baby continue. Treatment was continued and the baby survived. The little girl, Sharon Cutlass, is now sixteen months old and living at home with her parents.

The Cutlass family lives on a dairy farm about thirty-five miles from the hospital. I drove out to their home one afternoon to talk with them. Mainly I wanted to see how they were coping with the decision not to resuscitate a child who is now part of their family. Also, I wanted to explore the very real and strong emotions that parents have toward babies in the nursery as well as the role of human families in therapy decisions. The Cutlass house is white with blue shutters and is located directly across from their dark brown barn. Mrs. Cutlass came out to greet me when I arrived. Mr. Cutlass emerged from a shed wiping his hands. Their home is clean and sturdy with the hominess one finds in the Kansas of the *Wizard of Oz*. Mrs. Cutlass is an intelligent version of Auntie Em. During the interview their oldest son (who is four years old) made periodic appearances. They struck me as a strong and close family.

From an interview with Mr. and Mrs. Cutlass

Mrs. Cutlass: When Dr. Richmond took us into the nursery, our baby had had the bad [intracranial] bleeds that they knew were severe enough they could cause major problems or minor problems. I don't think they really know completely.

Mr. Cutlass: Well, they told us she was going to be a vegetable, in so many words.

Mrs. Cutlass: Dr. Wade told me that she had a hundred percent chance of being mentally or physically retarded.

Mr. Cutlass: Well now, one of them told us that she would not be able to eat, she would probably be blind and have to be fed through a tube for the rest of her life. At one point, we were told that. I can't tell you chronologically whether it was the first two days or two weeks or what, but we were told that. And it was very unlikely that they would be able to get her to suck a nipple.

Mrs. Cutlass: Unlikely she would have a sucking/swallowing reflex. But Dr. Richmond told us the first day that we went that there would come a time when she would have to go on a respirator. They were relatively sure. I think that was one of the worst, hardest decisions I've ever had to think about in my whole life—whether we wanted her to go on a respirator because of these bleeds. They were so severe that—what kind of a future would she have, and this type of thing. So we talked it over with Dr. Richmond and between ourselves and we made the decision that we didn't choose to. I think one of the problems was that we had never really had much contact with the doctors. The only time I had ever been in a hospital myself was to have the other children, and you consider a doctor to be completely knowledgeable. You put him on a pedestal. I've learned since not to, and I think it's wrong. But how else are you going to look at these people? Dr. Richmond is a person who has had a lot of experience in this type of field and you feel that she knows from her past experienes more or less what's going to happen. And Dr. Richmond agreed with our decision.

Mr. Cutlass: They said if it was their own children, that's what they would do. That's what Dr. Richmond said. It would be her decision—the same.

Mrs. Cutlass: So we more or less felt satisfied with the decision but when it came time that she was [to go] on a respirator, the decision was overruled by the hospital administration.

Mr. Cutlass: But see, the way we were looking at it, you have to understand, is that all they were doing was extending something that was inevitable. That's basically what we were told and what we believed, and we couldn't see our family, our whole family, grandparents and everything, everybody suffering along with her. That's the way we felt.

The hospital, in deciding that Sharon Cutlass was to be placed on a ventilator, broke longstanding precedents in ruling against its own staff and the parents of the child. Mr. and Mrs. Cutlass talked to their attorney about the possibility of legal action to force the hospital to cease aggressive treatment of their daughter. But, fearing unfavorable publicity for their family, they decided just to "drop it" and go along with the hospital's decision.

The Cutlasses explain the hospital decision mainly in terms of the administration's nervousness over lawsuits. The hospital's position (to their minds) was that parents are too distraught to make rational decisions on treatment for their babies and are liable to sue hospitals later if treatment is discontinued. A lawsuit of exactly this type had been brought in California shortly before the decision on the Cutlasses' daughter. The Cutlasses also heard that the hospital administration was concerned about the nursery staff—what the restrictions in therapy would do to the morale of those intimately caring for the babies. (My own research leads me to believe that this latter consideration is valid only if the nurses believe the baby has a real chance at survival, and there is no indication that they believed this in the case of the Cutlass baby.)

From the interview with Mr. and Mrs. Cutlass

Mrs. Cutlass: The type of problems she was going to have, we were just—the way we looked at it—prolonging her suffering, our suffering. I mean, that's part of it. I felt my mental state was part of it. She never actually had ever been our baby. Okay? We'd never held her. It wasn't like she had been home with us for a year or six months or something like this and then gotten critically ill and you were trying to save what love and life you had of her.

Mr. Cutlass: It was a strange feeling. It really was.

Mrs. Cutlass: It's really hard to understand.

Mr. Cutlass: Because she was up there so long that it almost was like two different worlds. We had to live with our kids and maintain our own lives as well as we could.

. . . . .

Frohock: And how is she now?

Mrs. Cutlass: She's a wild woman. (*Laughter.*) She's a joy. I guess the only way you could put it is that she's an ideal child. She's happy. She's content. She's a true addition to the family. When she came home before, when she had the colostomy and she was on this medication and that medication, she was so tiny—it was hard. It really was hard.

Frohock: You mentioned it was two worlds when she was in the hospital. Is it one world now?

Mr. Cutlass: Yes, she's part of the family and we're real happy to have her home. It looks like she's going to be pretty normal. I mean, what do you say? She's developed. Her muscle tone and all—that's good. She laughs and talks—not talks, but makes baby noises. She seems like a pretty much normal baby because her eyes flash around a bit. I don't know, maybe other babies do that also because they're always looking for something.

Mrs. Cutlass: Right. You're always worried with her if she doesn't eat when she's supposed to. Well, I'm not as bad as I used to be. If she doesn't finish her bottle, it's "Oh no, she's not going to gain weight." Instincts like this. But over a period of time you just kind of . . . She's gained weight so well and she hasn't always finished her bottle like she's supposed to. You kind of reinforce yourself that she's going to do all right this time.

Frohock: Looking back on that period of time in your lives when that crucial decision was made, do you have any thoughts on the certainty with which doctors can predict? Were they more wrong than right here?

Mr. Cutlass: I think they were. I think that there are a lot of people who may go up there that I'd like to talk to before they get too much of the doctors' advice. Whether we had a miracle or what we had—that it was really an exception is possible. But it just bothers me so much.

Frohock: What would you tell these people if you could talk to them?

Mr. Cutlass: I would tell them to fight it out a little bit more and not take the doctor's word at 100 percent.

. . . . .

Mr. Cutlass: I think it's hard for the doctors even to say something without being negative. How are you going to tell somebody your child's had a number 4 bleed without telling them what a number 4 bleed means? So then you've got to tell them the problems a number 4 bleed presents. And then you're involved with that and that's going through your mind. I guess everybody's different. Some people feel that a child like that should have—I don't want to say the right to live, because then it makes me feel like I'm saying I wanted to take away the right to live—but we just felt that she's got to have a respectable—I don't know, a right situation, enjoy life. I don't know. I've heard people say, "Well, how can you say that somebody that sits in a wheelchair is not enjoying life?" That's remote from this. But then you have to take that into perspective and say, "Yes, that's possible; that if I never could walk, I may well enjoy life in a wheelchair." But if you have a child that can't see, that can't move, that can't talk, that can't eat, it just seems like they can't possibly have any kind of life. That was the view that was being expressed by the doctors as a possibility.

Mrs. Cutlass: I think we would have felt differently, too, if it had been our first child. That's the way I feel. If it had been our first and we couldn't have any more—there are so many factors involved.

Mr. Cutlass: But you don't throw a child away just because you've got two others either. That's not what you mean.

Mrs. Cutlass: No, no. I guess that's not quite what I'm saying. We had children. We knew what it was like to have healthy, bouncy little babies and I guess I was being selfish. I didn't know what was entailed for me to take care of a child like that. I didn't know if I would be strong enough to do it. There's a lot involved. But I think we've all proved them wrong. It's something, I'll tell you.

. . . . .

Frohock: Who do you think ought to have the most effect on these decisions, the parents or the doctors?

Mr. Cutlass: No matter how you do it, the doctors are going to have the power basically. They're the ones who have the information and they have to be extremely careful how they present that. But yet you want the cards on the table too. You don't want any roses. But the parents should have the decision, definitely.

Mrs. Cutlass: I think that the doctors should tell the parents that everything that is humanly possible to keep their baby alive is going to be done. I didn't understand, really, what was going to go on. I had no idea.

. . . . .

Mr. Cutlass: It seems like they say things that are a little silly sometimes. Like one doctor says, "Well, she's such a bright-eyed, bushy-tailed little girl, she's got to make it." Well, what kind of an intelligent discussion are we having here? I mean, here she is—I don't remember what was going on at the time, probably a blood infection and some bowel problems, and we wanted him to do something. And he just off the cuff said that. It just seemed like that wasn't the way it ought to be handled. I mean, he meant well, I'm sure, by his statement.

At the end of the interview, Mrs. Cutlass brings Sharon into the living room. The baby is fresh from her nap and is blinking at the light. Her eyes, each of which has a detached retina, are abnormally large—wide and tall windows through which she sees. She is very small, looking more like six months than her age of sixteen months, and very lively. I take her from Mrs. Cutlass and hold her. She peers at me from exceedingly close range, seeming to study the things in front of her as one would scrutinize objects under a microscope. I cannot feel a trace of fear or nervousness in her. Her head jerks around as she looks with curiosity from object to object. It is impossible not to like her enormously. It is also not easy to think about refusing her a respirator when she was in need. Mr. Cutlass keeps referring to those days of decision. "The thought stays with me. It just sticks right up here in my head. I can't get rid of it." The no-code decision he and his wife made haunts him still.

At the opposite pole from the Cutlasses is Rita Monihan. Mrs. Monihan's baby, Jill, has been at Northeastern General for twenty-six months, for the past year in pediatrics. Every doctor I talked to is convinced that Jill has no chance for a recovery. She is a spina bifida victim who is severely brain-damaged, is on a respirator, has a colostomy, is blind from medication given to her during her last arrest, and continues to have periodic arrests (her heart stops beating) that bring her to the verge of death. Each time the hospital staff resuscitates Jill because Mrs. Monihan is adamant about continuing full treatment. The attending physicians advised her early on that her daughter's case is hopeless and that it would be best to forgo aggressive treatment when Jill arrests. Unlike Mr. and Mrs. Cutlass, however, Rita Monihan has insisted that aggressive therapy be continued.

Mrs. Monihan lives in a modest home on a country road almost ninety miles from Northeastern General. On the day I drove out to interview her, the weather was cold and clear. I tried to imagine how difficult it must be for her to get into the hospital to see Jill during the snow season. As I entered her home, a sizable group of family and friends walked out. Apparently there had been a conference about the interview before I arrived. Mrs. Monihan was friendly enough, confessing to me as I arranged the taping equipment that she was a bit nervous. I reassured her while trying to keep her cat away from the tape recorder. She told me before we began that Jill had broken her leg this morning at the hospital. Apparently the baby's bones are so brittle from not moving that they break very easily. Mrs. Monihan was composed during the interview, though not very articulate. There were glimpses of steel in her demeanor whenever she discussed her attitude toward treatment of her *daughter. Do every thing for her -- always.*

From an interview with Rita Monihan.

Mrs. Monihan: Well, when Jill was born—see, all the while I was pregnant with her, I was deadly sick. I went for a sonogram and everything—as far as I know, nothing showed up. But when she was born she had the spina bifida. And it was bad. So we took her out to Northeastern General. I didn't know what spina bifida was or anything. When I got out there and I saw her for myself, it was really bad. The doctors wanted to know what I wanted to do for her. I wanted them to do anything and everything they could do for her. Then they tell me about her outlook on life and everything, that her chances would never really be that good. They wanted to limit her medication and stuff. One at a time I told them no. I still wanted them to do everything that they could because my heart believed somehow something is going to come up to help her. Jill has spina bifida. She has hydrocephalus. She has many deformities. Her insides aren't where they're supposed to be. She has brain damage. She has the ileostomy bag on her for her bowels and right now she's taking medication that they gave her back in March. Even though she's that bad, she's gotten better in her own way. She isn't having all her spells. She was having seizures. She's not having all that now. And they have lowered her on her machinery, on the respirator. So I feel she is getting better even though she's not better. She may never be better, but to me, she's come that far. Considering the amount of times we've almost lost her and the time we did lose her and they brought her back, she has come a long way and I'm just not going to give up on her.

. . . . .

Frohock: Did you ever consider, at any time, not treating her fully when her arrests occurred?

Mrs. Monihan: No. I fought with several doctors over her because they—one doctor that I went to for myself, after Jill was born, told me I was a cruel mother, that I should never wish for my daughter to live. He really gave me a hard time. He was a good doctor—I liked him—but because of the things that he said, I wouldn't go back to him. Because she has as much right to live as anybody does. But every time I go out to Northeastern General they're always saying, "Are you sure you want us to do everything we can for her?" and I keep telling them over and over, yes. I want them just to do everything they can. It just about kills me every time they ask me that.

Then I had one of the doctors call me up one time—when she was born, they kept telling me that I should think of Jill. They kept calling me and telling me how bad she was and that I should think of what she's going through and everything. Well, a lot of things they said, I thought they were asking me to—that I should just let Jill go. So, one time they called me up, I had a friend of mine listen on the extension— you know, I thought maybe it was me—and my friend actually wanted to butt in on the line, she was so mad over what the doctor was telling me over the phone. And here I am standing there crying. I didn't want them telling me stuff like this. They said that she would never make it and she's made it this far.

Frohock: Did you ever think, before surgery, when that first deci-

sion was made whether to close the opening of the spine—
did you ever think then not to do it?

Mrs. Monihan: No, I didn't.

Frohock: Never?

Mrs. Monihan: No. When they called me and I was in the hospital,
the doctor said that they had to get her down to surgery
immediately. They wanted my permission over the phone.
Wanted to know if I wanted her to go to surgery or if I didn't.
You know, life or death. I told them that I definitely wanted
her to go. Do anything and everything they could do for her.
Even though it was so bad the doctor said that she may not
even pull through it, I still wanted them to do it. As you can
see, she pulled through it. She pulled through it several
times.

Frohock: A lot of people are afraid of doctors. How did you come to
take control of your child's destiny?

Mrs. Monihan: Well, when I was in the hospital and Jill was out
there and they called, said it was either life or death if they
didn't take her to surgery, I just let them do it. I knew when
she went through the surgery once and she pulled through it,
and she had to go as many times as she did after, I figured if
they helped her once, they're going to help her again. Every
time anything's ever come up about her, I've just got my faith
in the doctor. So I don't know. Because I'm afraid of doctors
myself. I always was.

Frohock: Suppose a doctor came up to you and said, "We should
stop treatment." What would you say to that doctor?

Mrs. Monihan: No.

Frohock: So you will stand up to them?

Mrs. Monihan: Yeah. If they say that, I sure would.

Two cases. One in which the parents accepted the do-not-
resuscitate advice of their doctors, and then, because of a very
unusual and surprising intervention by the hospital administration,
their baby was treated and survived. The other in which the parents
opposed the do-not-resuscitate advice of their doctors and now
have a severely damaged child. Both parents believe in miracles, the
first because a miracle happened and the second because the mother
wants a miracle to happen. What is the lesson to be learned from
these experiences? One is that doctors are sometimes wrong and
that doctors are sometimes right. And that the hospital system for
making decisions on therapy is not fail-safe.

3

April 3. Stephanie is sleeping on her right side, her left hand covering her ear as if shutting out sound. Her abdomen is swollen, red. Both of her legs are now swathed in the biobrane. It looks like white knit stockings. She is breathing rapidly. A toy zoo is at the top of her bed. Nearby is a pile of medical instruments next to a small, flat, toy kitten. The thermometer hanging from a shelf in her room reads 95°. Her parents are here. The mother is slowly slowly putting on her isolation garb looking like she has just been crying. The father is restless, pacing about in the halls. A very large nurse is in with Stephanie at the moment—a bulky figure wrapped in a blue gown, net over her hair, light blue mask on. She is moving slowly as she goes about her tasks, a well-balanced figure who appears to be floating gently under water over some flat surface.

There is very little uncertainty among the group of individuals—the parents and staff—who have decided not to try heroic measures on Stephanie. They know now she is not going to survive.

As I leave the nursery for the day I stop by Stephanie's room and look at her again through the window. Her left arm seems separated from her body by a deep lesion. She is covered by red welts. The biobrane knit stocking has slid up past her thighs.

April 4. For a change of pace and in order to see some graduates of the nursery who have made it past pediatrics and are living at home, I spend the day at the spina bifida clinic in the hospital.

Two children stand out from the group, though for different reasons. One is a twelve-year-old boy, Ken, whose legs are withered and whose speech is severely impaired. He communicates with his mother by grunts and facial expressions that he can vary skillfully. He seems to size up situations in the examination room quite well and expresses his feelings by groans and smiles. He and his mother are very affectionate with each other, exchanging many kisses and sidelong glances. There is more than a fair amount of mischief in this boy. The mother is very concerned about his schooling. It seems that her son tries to kiss those schoolmates he likes, and he effectively ignores those he dislikes. This pattern of affection and exclusion unsettles the school officials, who apparently cannot understand that a handicapped child, one who is restricted in movement and communication, may yet have strong and normal emotions. Ken progressed well in normal classes, but because of his emotional responses he has been placed in a class of handicapped children. There, according to his mother, he is regressing intellectually. The school officials have told his mother that "there is no school for Ken." This attitude understandably infuriates Ken's mother, though she won't raise too loud a protest for fear that Ken will be removed from the school.

The second child is a beautiful blond boy, Jeremy, only three and one-half years old, an obvious joy to his parents. He starts flirting with me immediately. The therapist is checking his cognitive development with manual tests. Jeremy stacks blocks with ease. He draws a straight line on request. The therapist draws a circle and asks him to draw one. He says, "Face," and fills in the therapist's circle with eyes, nose, mouth. The general check of his coordination goes well. He has some problems touching his left thumb to his left fingers. The therapist balances him on a rocker. Suddenly he loses his balance and falls backward. His father catches his head before it strikes the floor. Incredible, but this child has come very close to serious injury in an accidental fall in the hospital. He is lucky—in several respects.

It is true what they say. Bad things do happen to good people. One is reminded of the Greek sense of tragedy—individuals of character finding themselves in tragic situations because of the contradictions of life. The very decency of some of the parents in the nursery leads to the painful results that weaker or more self-interested individuals might avoid. Ken's mother is a dedicated woman who would do anything for her son. Her life will probably be spent in caring for Ken. The parents of Jeremy have another child with a mild case of cerebral palsy. They are intelligent and loving parents, coping very well with what they have—indeed, thriving as a family. They have enveloped the two events in their lives with a general affirmation of life. They turn the bad into good. They are also lucky that their children have only mild problems.

Two observations are worth mentioning. The first is that asking if the children in the spina bifida clinic are human is absurd and insulting. They are as human as you or I. Humanness is not the issue. The second is that family response is a key variable in predicting how a baby will fare. And this variable is unpredictable. The staff at the hospital tell me again and again how difficult it is to read a family. You never know, they say, which families will love and work with their handicapped children. The conclusion that follows this second observation is important. Even if reliable correlations existed between the physical condition of a spina bifida baby and later development of the child (and such correlations do not exist), the unknown variable of family response would still make prognosis very uncertain.

I stop by the nursery before leaving the hospital to look in on Stephanie. She is lethargic, her nurse tells me, not "raising hell" anymore. A bad sign. Her left arm is now also (in addition to her legs) enveloped in the biobrane. She is sleeping on her left side, a strip of vaseline-soaked paper extending down her back. Two doctors are in her room along with her nurse. Her abdomen seems even more distended today. One doctor picks up a brown paper bag and takes out sterile gauze (oblivious to the fact that he has just broken the sterilization of the gloves). This doctor is now gently swabbing a pink fluid on Stephanie's right arm inside of her elbow where there is a raw abrasion. Stephanie twists in pain, crying. He places a light gauze on the wound, winding it around her arm. Now he adds several more layers of gauze. On top of the gauze he places a strip of biobrane (the knitlike covering). Stephanie turns. She is in agony. I can now see how terribly swollen and inflamed her abdomen is. She is starting to resemble the ghastly photographs of starving children with bloated abdomens. Except she has also been through a fire.

Can some component of the self—the will to live or maybe the soul itself—still be intact and rail against the ravages of the body? I am becoming a believer again in the doctrine of dualism. Stephanie's spirit is separate and fighting against the conditions of her body.

4

The problem in defining human beings may be that the relevant terms are not fixed but open and variable. The definitions try to meet impossible requirements: that something distinctive about human existence can be identified and isolated; that this special something extends to all human beings, no matter what their condition, and that no other living creatures are caught by the criteria; and that the special something is constant across all moral and scientific theories (that no matter what else we believe, self-definitions remain the same). No definition of human beings will meet these tests beyond the simple fact of unique chromosomal arrangements, and chromosomes do not express anything about our human capacities to think, love, and work.

Perhaps the method of defining is wrong. There may be no

unique test of humanness. Being human may in itself mean being the source and object of multiple definitions, each of which may vary with shifts in moral perspective. Consider the children in the nursery. They are all human beings, regardless of their condition. By this I mean that, within the practice of medicine, they are *regarded* as human beings. Outside of the nursery, or within the nursery among those babies the staff has decided at the beginning not to treat, the designation of human is not clear or indisputable. Even the language is qualified. "Fetus," for example, is the most commonly used term to refer to those infants too premature to admit or treat. Yet the main difference between such infants and those admitted for treatment is viability. If an infant is not going to survive, he is outside the practice of neonatology. We might even say he has failed a membership test, and in failing the test he is excluded from a community of human skills—even though he may pass tests set by other human communities.

Suppose we dismiss the thought that there is one definition of human beings everywhere. Perhaps the beginning and end of our humanness is with the communities to which we belong. For an infant to count as a member of the nursery (as a human community) he must be able to make it, survive. This is the primal function that specifies membership. To be a member of a religious community, however, an infant must simply be (a) born, or (b) conceived—depending on the type of religious community. Neonatology is not the art or science of spiritual salvation. The practice of religion is. The two communities are opposed on tests for entry into a human community.

Much of the agony of parents can be explained as a conflict among different human communities. The Cutlasses and the Monihans are caught between competing social practices. One, drawn from religious or natural right philosophers, and perhaps also from the imperatives of family life itself, fixes the values of individuals in absolute terms. Each person is given a unique and overriding value. The other is the practice of neonatology, where individuals are evaluated in viability terms. No universally accepted principles fuse or order these practices. How can an absolute value be compromised by a feasibility measure like survival? The absolute value says, do everything (or you will suffer remorse). The feasibility value says, do only what is sensible. And so the Cutlasses and the Monihans are torn between peremptory and practical imperatives, each of which is rational in terms of the domains of different human communities. If a simple and universal definition of humanness existed, the Cutlasses and the Monihans would not be pulled in opposite rational directions.

Multiple definitions of humanness, when joined to the uncertainty found in early prognosis, suggest that decisions on treatment must have an open or indeterminate form. What weights to assign to quality-of-life considerations, and even how to order these considerations, depends on the importance assigned to different human communities. And, since there seems to be nothing available to rank the communities, parents and physicians are free to make therapy decisions without violating some determinate and universal sense of humanness. Pain and guilt, rather than immorality and irrationality, plague therapy decisions. And much of this distress is explained by the closeness of community members, where grief for a stricken associate is one mark of community ties. An especially compelling form of association is the family. Even here, however, several understandings of humanness compete for attention when hard cases must be decided.

The hardest case on the nursery floor at the moment is Stephanie Christopher. At the moment her interests have been adjusted to exclude emergency resuscitation. No one sees any point in summoning her back from the grave to continue the pain she suffers. She is a human without prospects. All communities represented in the nursery know that by now, though it is still hard for the family and some of the staff to accept it.

7
Law and Medicine

1

April 5. Stephanie's sodium level is very low. She is also bleeding now consistently through her stool and urine, not intermittently as before. The nurse says she weeps more from her lesions. Her platelet count is low, below 50,000 now in spite of platelet transfusions. She has rubbed off all of the skin from the top of the forefinger of her left hand, where the skin is curling down now and hanging like a clear bandaid. The biobrane covering has now been extended by the staff to cover her upper torso. It is so hot in her room that nurses are now spending only thirty minutes inside at a time before coming out to keep watch on Stephanie through her window.

A newly installed television set in the hall is showing a closed-circuit program on the biobrane dressings now being used on Stephanie. The patients in the demonstration program are all burn victims. A nurse yesterday asked why all of Stephanie's skin could not be treated at once with the biobrane. But apparently the substance works only on lesions. The dressings, as a kind of skin surrogate, are supposed to decrease pain as well as promote healing. The nurses are very attentive during the TV presentation.

Danielle Raymond is improving. She is breathing only with a hood, no ventilator. The Blackwell baby is awake, still undiagnosed and staring without blinking at what looks like a connection for a CPAP.

April 6. Stephanie had a seizure this morning. She just stopped breathing. The staff brought her out of it by holding the oxygen mask directly to her face and by stimulating her manually (shaking her body, as if waking someone up). She is sleeping at the moment, the oxygen mask still near her face and blowing air directly on her.

She turns blue now whenever the oxygen is turned off. She may be septic and is currently receiving antibiotics. Stephanie's nurse says, "She took a long time coming back this morning." The nurse called the attending physician at his home when the breathing problems began. He immediately put her on the defensive. "Why call me? She isn't arresting." The nurse agrees with the no-resuscitation order in Stephanie's chart. "There is no point to intubation. She'll still only get worse. She'll die of sepsis, even with antibiotics prolonging the end. Unless her line gets infected. Then it'll be quicker."

I run into Randy Hunter in the hall. I ask him how the talk went with Stephanie's parents. "I simply said to them," he tells me with a perfect poker face, "that I planned to stop all therapy and let the kid croak. But if they wanted to prolong the dying by insisting on an I.V., that was up to them." I ask how the parents responded to this sensitive and caring way of presenting the problem. "Actually—the true story is that I explained the options to them, what we were doing and why. The father said, uh huh, uh uh, and then left. The mother asked questions about the treatment—why didn't we do this instead of that, and so on."

Hunter is getting ready to present his slide show on accidental injuries to babies in the nursery—bruised newly borns (from forceps, for example), babies accidentally burned by monitoring equipment, I.V. problems, etc. Hunter is convinced that such accidents can be avoided. I notice that all of the doctors going into his conference room are eating junk foods—chocolate covered popsicles, ice cream sandwiches, cones replete with chemical nuts. So much for physicians as role models for dietary habits.

The staff is keeping Stephanie on 30 percent oxygen, which seems to allow her to hold her own and breath normally.

Some thoughts. One standard, the best interests of the child, and one rule, substituted judgment, are used in deciding on treatment for infants. All physicians and nurses believe that the child's best interests ought to prevail in therapy decisions, not the "humanness" of the baby (whatever that means). To express these interests they try to reconstruct what the child would choose for herself if she were a competent adult. It is interesting that the standard and the rule can compete with each other at the adult level. A valid living will, for example, can be used to state what a comatose adult would choose in the way of therapy. A best-interests standard might select a different therapy. If the revealed preference is not too eccentric, one supposes that the patient has his way against a best-interests choice. But there is still uncertainty about how to use substituted judgment in the case of infant children, who have no living wills, no life from which to infer what a choice would be. What does substituted judgment draw upon to settle choices on therapy? Perhaps a more generalizable best-interests standard would provide the values in stipulating what any competent person would choose as therapy. In this case, quality of life must be used to flesh out the interests. Or perhaps one can construct particular best interests for an infant by combining, through some weighting system, a cluster of physical condition and prognosis (including the factor of uncertainty); (b) mental abilities, pain, longevity, mobility, morphology; (c) family context, including the attitudes of relevant figures in the family as well as the existence or not of other children; and (d) institutional support (in part as a substitute for family support). Perhaps a kind of scientific horoscope can be made up for each child as a basis for identifying the child's best interests.

April 8. Stephanie looks ghastly. The biobrane experiment has failed. Her skin has not improved with the treatment and, in fact, the gauze needed to hold the dressings on her skin caused even more abrasions. It is disheartening. Everyone—surgeons, dermatologists, and burn experts—had been hopeful that the biobrane treatment would bring some relief and help stabilize her condition. It has not. The doctors have gone back to the older more standard treatment—gauzes socked in vaseline. Stephanie's legs, arms, abdomen have deep red gashes with caked blood on them. She is breathing rapidly, her face a few inches away from the oxygen mask. She looks like an accident victim—tired, even worn out, from some disaster that has struck her. What looks like the remains of one of the biobrane dressings is sticking to her elbow. Stephanie's mother calls. She wants an update on her daughter's condition. But the nurse caring for Stephanie is downstairs at lunch.

A mother is here. She is a teenager, overweight and exhausted, pimples covering her face. A child who has just given birth to a child. Cindy Blackwell is on CPAP, covered with a cotton blanket. She opens her eyes, rolls them up, goes back to sleep. A sign, "Wash your hands, drown a germ," hangs from the wall of room A.

A small boy, about four years old, has come to the nursery with his parents and grandmother to see his younger sister. The sister is a premature baby, as he was some years ago here in this same nursery. He suffers from cerebral palsy. The parents hold the baby up to the window so that the boy and his grandmother can see her from the hall (since only parents are allowed in the rooms). One of the older nurses is in tears in a private moment by herself in a corner of the hall. Later she tells us that she had cared for the boy when he was a baby in the nursery.

In Stephanie's room, in the same wing where the visit is taking place, a nurse is taking Stephanie's temperature by placing a thermometer in her arm pit. Then the nurse replaces the vaseline gauzes on her body. Stephanie is crying as the gauzes are removed. Her left leg is bloody, her foot scraped raw over the ankle and on top. Her right leg looks better except for a large lesion with a scab under the area of the knee. Some of the gauzes are soaked with blood. Her hands are also bloody.

Across the hall the visiting parents and grandmother are admiring the long eyelashes the boy and his sister have.

The world is truly anomalous. Things do *not* fit together. Yesterday my younger daughter won first prize in a mathematics symposium. Stephanie will not win anything. Is the point to her life the effects she is having on others? Then what are these effects and where is the structure of events in which these effects can be located?

Stephanie is getting morphine now in regular and heavy doses.

One can look at individuals in either of two ways. On one view individual life is an egoistic time span of benefit primarily to the individual who lives the life. On the other, individuals are constituent members of a social unit which has as one of its features the belief that individuals exist as much for the sake of others as for themselves. Do therapy decisions differ as one adopts one of these views or the other?

April 9. A new baby is in the intensive wing. She is being examined by Joe Ritiglia. Her eyes are open but, in Ritiglia's words, "she is not tracking." The nurse helping him says, "The lights are on, but no one's at home." Ritiglia: "Exactly."

A nurse is massaging a baby's chest with an electric rubber plunger that goes up and down very rapidly. Looks like fun, though it is a serious effort to clear his bronchial tubes. In another part of the same room Danielle Raymond's mother sits vacantly by her baby's bed.

Stephanie's nurse, whoever it may be, now sits outside her room looking through the window at Stephanie most of the time.

2

The Baby Doe case on Long Island is in the news again. Two days ago the parents of the little girl, whose name is Keri-Lynn, announced that they had brought their daughter home from the hospital. They said that the opening in her spine had healed on its own without surgery. The lower portions of Keri-Lynn's legs are paralyzed. But the parents were convinced that surgery would have caused even more problems, including permanent nerve damage. They also revealed that they had persuaded doctors to insert a shunt in Keri-Lynn's brain to drain fluid to her abdomen. This surgery, performed three weeks ago, relieved pressure on the child's brain and allowed Keri-Lynn to leave the hospital. The parents were critical of their legal opponents, remarking that the natural healing of Keri-Lynn's meningomyelocele made a "joke" of the legal attempts to mandate surgery. Critics pointed out, however, that the spinal opening always heals naturally without surgery, and that the point of the surgery is to prevent infection. There was a report that Keri-Lynn did have an infection at one time, though no information was ever released on how serious the infection was. Also, some doctors (at other hospitals) pointed out that the shunt is most effective in preventing brain damage if implanted immediately after birth.

At the time of this news, with exquisite timing, Lawrence Washburn appears on my campus. He is the right-to-life attorney who initiated the lawsuit against Keri-Lynn's parents. Apparently he is speaking in various areas of the country to air his views and continue the discussion of these issues at public forums. His position, expressed in both speaking engagements (sometimes in tandem with the attorney representing Keri-Lynn's parents, Paul Gianelli— a kind of soft-shoe dance through the issues by the adversaries) and in articles, is a curious mix of substance and procedure.

The substance is flint-hard. Washburn believes, along with many others in the right-to-life movement, that all human life ought to be maintained no matter what its quality. There is no reason to think that he would prolong dying in hopeless cases, for many in the pro-life movement (Nat Hentoff, for example) would not sanction intervention to resuscitate a person who will live only for a short time before inevitably dying. But Washburn and others believe that the quality of an infant's life (except perhaps at very high thresholds—say, an anencephalic baby) should not be a consideration in therapy decisions. Or, put in Washburn's language, that an infant is handicapped is irrelevant in treating the infant.

The procedure is more subtle. Washburn maintains that decisions on therapy for infant children are flawed in one vital respect: no one represents the interests of the child. He argues that (a) a child needs a disinterested guardian as her representative, and (b) an evidentiary proceeding is needed to confirm medical diagnosis and review treatment decisions. Washburn claims further that decisions not to treat babies with severe defects are in violation of federal laws prohibiting discrimination against handicapped persons. His brief against the parents of Keri-Lynn represented all of these points. He stressed in later accounts of the case that no one—parents, physicians, hospital—had asserted the child's individual rights to personal security and equal medical care and treatment in a state institution. The parents had exercised the power of substituted judgment for their child without a judicial review of this judgment. His efforts were designed to provide such review in the courts.

Washburn's brief is a challenge to well-established practices. By law and tradition the parents and the physicians are regarded as the child's proper surrogates. Privacy is normally accorded to therapy decisions unless a legal challenge is made by one of the interested parties (parents or physicians) to a decision. The current procedure in the nursery has one built-in safeguard that inclines decisions toward, rather than away from, aggressive therapy. If *any* interested party—parent or physician—want the child treated, the child is treated. Sometimes, as with Jill Monihan, the result is an apparent overtreatment with results that, in the opinion of everyone but the mother, are not in the child's best interests. On occasion the system fails to treat those who should be treated. Sharon Cutlass is an example. A charitable critic might say the hospital administration saved the system in the Cutlass case by mandating treatment. But such an intervention is so unusual that it cannot be counted as part of a fail-safe system. If the usual procedures had been followed, Sharon Cutlass would now be dead instead of living at home with her parents. Washburn seems to feel that the procedures on therapy decisions are inherently, not occasionally, defective *against* therapy, and that an additional champion of the child must be appointed from outside the system. He is trying to change radically a practice supported for centuries as the best way to decide on medical treatment for children.

Several questions are raised by Washburn's campaign. One is what will happen to the procedural part of the program if substance and procedure conflict with each other. The guiding principle of his reform effort is the sanctity of human life. The procedural part of the program is designed to guarantee that principle on the assumption that current procedures fail the principle in the area of neonatology. But suppose the reform procedures are put in place—a disinterested guardian for the child and evidentiary proceedings in law—and the new arrangements lead to a fresh emphasis on quality of life against maintaining life? Suppose the reforms result in more rather than fewer decisions not to treat defective newborns?

The connection between substance and procedure is notoriously devious. Law is hardly free of such complexity. Right-to-life attorneys will recall that the courts, at the highest levels, liberalized abortion practices in the United States. Because of such court decisions the right-to-life movement has turned to legislatures to safeguard the life of what they see as an unborn child. Pro-choice supporters, by contrast, favor legal over legislative action on abortion issues (for equally obvious reasons). Each side supports a different procedure because of substantive commitments. If procedures fail to realize cherished principles, and the procedures are endorsed precisely to implement the principles, then the program has failed at the deepest level. One can reasonably expect the rejection of procedure—on principled grounds. It would be neither surprising nor irrational for Washburn and his supporters to abandon the procedural part of their program if the procedures do not guarantee right-to-life principles in treating defective newborns. Then the question is—what procedures will replace legal review?

A second question is raised by the use of "handicaps" in Washburn's program. Washburn seems to use the term in a generic sense—as referring to any physical liability. Keri-Lynn's handicaps included hydrocephalus, microcephalus, and spina bifida. But the notion of a handicap that includes sush a range of conditions can also include debilities that justify *not* treating infants. It is, in general, a handicap (as the term is used in Washburn's suit) to be born at twenty-five weeks' gestation with a body weight of under 500 grams. Such babies are, on the whole, nonviable—surely a severe handicap. It is also a handicap to have trisomy 13 or 18, or to be born without a brain. Yet these are precisely the types of extreme physical conditions that warrant less aggressive therapy *because* of the "handicap." To say, as Washburn says, that a handicap can never be a relevant consideration in treatment decisions requires that we have a more refined definition of "handicap" than currently provided.

Perhaps the most important question, however, is drawn from the relationship between law and medicine. Can legal proceedings adequately supervise medical decisions? The two social practices differ in critical ways. Neonatology, like all forms of medical practice, is a cooperative enterprise in which consultation among practitioners is vital to success. Physicians in the nursery need information and use their colleagues to get it. Doctors may try to tough it out with individual diagnoses in other areas of medicine. But teams of doctors in the nursery routinely provide different insights and perspectives on medical problems. The contrast with law is sharp. Legal proceedings are adversarial. Attorneys oppose one another in a contest with winners and losers. Truth is disclosed (ideally) in a conflict regulated closely by rules of evidence and inference. The cooperative features of medicine are at the opposite extreme from the rules and expectations of legal proceedings.

Medical decisions are also different from legal decisions. Therapy decisions are serial and remedial. They proceed stepwise, with frequent incremental revisions as information is updated. There are few final decisions in neonatology. Even decisions not to treat are reversible if conditions warrant. Stephanie, for example, is currently a qualified no-code baby (do not resuscitate with a ventilator). But these instructions would be changed quickly if her ability to cope with her skin disease improved. Therapy decisions in the nursery are also tentative, based on imperfect information. The public image of the physician as god is not confirmed by observations in the nursery, where doctors are readily aware both of their limitations and of the complexities of diagnosis at the early stages of life. Therapy decisions are always part of a continual process of monitoring patients and revising judgments.

Legal decisions, especially those that culminate a legal proceeding, are singular and decisive. Law is, of course, a social practice in which decisions typically modify and extend earlier precedents. But nothing in the nursery parallels the finding or verdict at the end of a hearing or trial. Such decisions close inquiries. Law admits continuations, of course. Decisions can be appealed (endlessly, it sometimes seems), and some decisions establish a series of decisions. Bankruptcy proceedings, for example, are court-ordered efforts to monitor over time the dissolution of a business or the settlement of an individual's liabilities. But the decision made by a jury or judge can also decisively conclude legal activities (akin, one supposes, to a death in medicine). Such decisions are also not tentative. They frequently establish precedents and determine guilt or innocence.

The very languages of medicine and law are unlike one another. Patients are not defendants. No one in medicine is charged with an offense, or presumed innocent (or found guilty) in the nursery. The patients are outside the pale of all responsibility-assigning languages. They are simply ill children. Perhaps the greatest difference in language, however, is found in a term common to both medical and legal practice—"interest." Therapy decisions are focused on special interests. These interests are brought into the nursery by the infants and families. The physicians resist generalizing particular interests. They constantly claim that there are no standard interests that cut across the variety of situations they face. Each case, they say, has unique features that require special handling. Law, by contrast, addresses objective or general interests. Legal cases always involve persons, and courts address the particular facts of cases (including the intentions and motives of individuals.) But courts also ensure that individuals fit legal categories. Ultimately individuals are seen in law not as particular persons, but as members of classes of persons recognized by legal rules. The power and virtue of law are in its eventual subordination of particular cases to rules for treating different individuals in like fashion.

Washburn's proposals introduce the logic of law into medical practice—disinterestedness, adversarial proceedings, conclusive decisions, objective interests, and even rights. It is not easy to see how a legal hearing can remain consistent with the special commitments, consultative and cooperative actions, serial and tentative decisions, and particularized interests of neonatology. Reform by its nature intends to change the object of its attention to something better. But it is important to understand how much of medical practice will be changed if therapy decisions are governed by judicial review.

3

April 10. Danielle Raymond is doing very well. She has only a hood now over her head to supply her with oxygen. The CPAP has been removed. Across from her bed, Randy Hunter is overseeing an intern's attempt to change intubation tubes on a baby. The intern is working silently, a small bead of perspiration slowly working its way down his left cheek. "Talk to me, George," Hunter says. "I can't help you if you don't talk to me." The intern is squinting down an instrument inserted into the baby's throat. "I think the new line is in place." "Then pull the old line out," Hunter replies, "and slip the new one in with one motion." The intern moves his hands back and forth. "It worked. It's in." He sounds surprised. Hunter strolls off: "Way to go, George. You just saved another life."

Stephanie is wrapped in what looks like a shroud of white vaseline. Her hands seem to hold the oxygen mask a few inches from her face. The stream of oxygen is pouring straight into her eyes, nose, mouth. The bed surface constantly flutters from the hot air blown upward to hold the spheres aloft. The nurse is outside the room seated in a chair near the window overlooking Stephanie's bed. She is reading a novel.

The attending physicians are still trying to keep Stephanie's electrolytes in balance and maintain a proper level of bodily fluids. She is not gaining weight despite the maximum amounts of sugar, fat and protein being pumped into her. The staff has twice attempted parenteral feeds (intraveneously) in April, but the result in each case was massive stool output and some intestinal bleeding. Stephanie will just not tolerate any feedings, and her caloric intake is still being (imperfectly) met with fluids, sugar, and electrolytes. Her skin lesions are not more numerous (though it sometimes seems so in looking at her), but her blood platelet level is still low and the lesions constantly ooze blood. She has been treated with antibiotics off and on as a precaution, though only one blood culture has been positive (for an infection). Her condition, given the disease from which she suffers, is considered stable at the present time.

A mother of one of the babies in the nursery comes over and complains to the nurses at the desk that another outfit belonging to her baby has been lost. One of the nurses goes back with her into the rooms to search for it. Another nurse holds her chest and forehead and cries out dramatically, "We've done it again." One of the older nurses tells a story about one mother who went to the hospital administration to complain about the loss of a pink elephant. The nurses are bemused over these happenings.

One of the nurses in the level 1 wing comes over to Randy Hunter and tells him at length how one of the doctors (the same doctor who accosted me in the hall back at the beginning of my study) shouted at her for telling some parents something erroneous about their baby's treatment. The end of the story is that this doctor then later came over to her and quietly apologized. The nurse, however, is still angry and somewhat apprehensive, for during the "apology" the doctor shouted at her again about something.

April 11. Stephanie's head is damp with sweat. The rest of her body, her entire torso, is covered in vaseline-soaked gauzes. She seems to be bleeding from her upper buttocks. The nurse is in her room and very attentive: checking Stephanie's heart with a stethoscope, watching her, checking the oxygen indicators, and so on. Blood keeps soaking through the bandages in the area of Stephanie's lower back. The nurse carefully places two identical cat dolls on the bed above Stephanie's head.

Danielle Raymond looks better every time I see her. She is still using a hood for oxygen and she still has episodes of apnea and bradycardia (a slowing of the heart rate). But her color and general body tone seem much better. The oxygen hood currently in Danielle's bed is the size of a small cage. Danielle is sleeping on her stomach with practically her whole body inside the hood. The hood, enveloped in cellophane, is partially opaque. A large, pink, Big Bird doll is on Danielle's bed outside the hood, pointed toward her face.

A baby on the side of the room where Danielle Raymond is located has presented an interesting problem lately for the staff to ponder. The baby has a normal brain and is generally doing well with one critical exception. He was born prematurely, had to be put immediately on a respirator, and his lungs are currently, in the words of the staff, "shot all to hell." The respirator is his respiratory organ. Is he to be kept for the rest of his life on a tube inserted from his throat into his lungs? Is a life of artificial, machine-driven respiration a worthwhile life? These are the same questions pondered at the beginning of my study, and the staff confronts them again and again without answers.

Cindy Blackwell remains the mystery baby. In spite of numerous consultations with specialists, including especially neurologists, her condition has not been diagnosed. She is being treated as if a brain dysfunction exists in the lower limbic area of the brain. But no one knows anything about her true condition, only that she has potentially life-threatening symptoms of apnea. There is some talk about sending her to Chicago to be examined and treated by physicians who are recognized as the best in treating this general species of disorder. At the moment she is propped up in an infant seat with a white bandage around her head where an I.V. is inserted in a scalp vein. The white bandage gives her a kind of jaunty look, though the I.V. reminds one of the gravity of her condition. A ventilator tube is in her mouth. A nurse injects a dark fluid into the I.V. leading into her scalp. Anyone still believing in the universal miracles of modern medicine is quickly brought back to reality in confronting the genuine puzzlement of doctors treating this baby.

Rebecca Smith, the nurse who first handled Stephanie, is now working in the opposite wing of the nursery treating other babies. She has just discovered that she is pregnant. This discovery led her to ask out of the rotation on Stephanie. The request was granted. She says it was fortunate because she couldn't have done it much longer anyway. "Too hot. And one thing I've always known is that I couldn't treat burn patients." And of course Stephanie is a burn patient who keeps burning up every day.

There are two nurses in front of Stephanie's room trading information. One is replacing the other. The nurse who has completed her stay with Stephanie is saying, "She's congested, spitting up phlegm. But I don't want to suction her because blood comes up. Her whole mouth is shedding inside." She takes off the sterile gown. "She likes the oxygen. She really didn't like it when we had to move her to draw blood. She wants that mask." One of the doctors had difficulty earlier in finding an artery to draw blood. "Maybe she's leaving," the new nurse says. "And maybe she's not," the other nurse responds.

April 12. Stephanie's lower back is full of blood. Red-soaked gauzes cover the area. Her mother is here. She is talking to another woman who is visiting the nursery with her. "Stephanie is even smaller than Katy." (Katy is the earlier daughter who died of the same disease.) There is a report circulating in the hospital that Stephanie's mother broke down this past weekend and rescinded the no-resuscitation order. On Monday, after again talking to the doctors, she is said to have reinstated the order. Stephanie's treatment continues to be antibiotics when needed, transfusions, oxygen, and burn therapy—but no CPR if she arrests.

> *From an interview with Stephanie's parents conducted four months after the observations in the hospital. Mr. and Mrs. Christopher have a house in a trailer park in a small village fifty-five miles from Northeastern General. They are both obviously affected by Stephanie's sufferings, but Mrs. Christopher is the more articulate of the*

two. She speaks in moving tones about Stephanie, and breaks down at one point in the interview.

Frohock: Now, at one point in the treatment, you and the doctors sat down and made a decision not to intubate Stephanie.

Mrs. Christopher: Well, that scared me. Bill [her husband] was home when this happened. Dr. Sanchez [the dermatologist] was sitting there and I asked him how she was doing. He says "Well, we have to make a decision." The way he put it, or the way he said it, and the way I took it was that he was telling me that I had to decide whether or not she should live or die. I didn't understand exactly what he was saying and it really scared me. So I called Bill and I told him. I said, "I don't know what to do." Then it wasn't too long after that I saw Dr. West. I asked him what it was they were telling me. He told me that if she had gone into heart failure, where her heart stopped, whether or not I would want him to bring her back and put her on a respirator. I said, "Well, what do you suggest?" and he said "Well, if it was me, I wouldn't because of the chance of brain damage." And just knowing that they'd have to press on her chest to get her heart going again, or whatever they had to do, they'd probably do more damage to her than if they were just to leave her alone. And I told him, "Well, if that happens, let her be." I talked to Bill first and I said, "Well, if it's going to happen, it's going to happen and there's nothing we can do about it because a respirator is only going to keep her heart pumping." She can die and her heart's going to—the machine's going to keep going, but she's not there. I said, "Well, if it happens, let her be. There's nothing we're going to be able to do about it anyway, because when she's gone, that's it.

Mr. Christopher: We knew pretty much that she was going to die.

Mrs. Christopher: We knew she was going to die, but we just didn't know when and gradually she got weaker. Betsy Randolph, one of the older nurses there that took care of her, would sit down with me. We'd talk and she told me that eventually Stephanie was going to say, "I'm tired. I want to go to sleep," and that'd be it. I figured, "Well, she's going to die. I know that." But we weren't sure when it was going to happen, because she was doing real good for a while.

Frohock: Did you ever rethink that decision not to intubate, and change your mind in the weeks or so following it?

Mrs. Christopher: No. Because we knew that if we did that, we'd be doing more damage to her. It would only be postponing what should have happened. It would be dragging it out, making her suffer more. That's what hurt us the most. Because we'd sit and we'd look at her and I'd go in—it was so hot in there. Bill couldn't go in for very long. It was between 94 and 97 degrees and on top of everything that we had to put on, it was just unbearable in there. He can't stand the heat anyway. So he'd only stay in five, maybe ten minutes, maybe a little longer and then he'd come back out. But I could go in and I could stay in there half an hour, forty-five minutes. It didn't bother me because I was putting all my attention on her. I couldn't pick her up. I couldn't really do anything with her, except that her head was so small that I could just gradually rub my hand over it and I'd calm her down so quick. Because she'd cry, and that really bothered us. We'd sit there and we'd watch her cry and I couldn't stand to watch her cry. So the minute I saw her crying, I'd get right up and I'd go right in to quiet her down. Because she'd cry and then she'd kick her bandages right off and do a lot of damage to her body.

Mrs. Christopher's tenderness toward Stephanie is unusual in the nursery. The main affection these babies get is from the nurses. They rock the babies, kiss them and cuddle them, talk to them—while the latest in technology extends from the babies' bodies. Mary Jane Kennedy is rocking baby Julia Allen to sleep at this moment, the intubation tube connected to Julia's nose and mouth. Julia has been in the nursery four months. Her lungs are severely damaged. She may also have some neurological problems. Kennedy plays hide-and-seek with this unconscious baby, calling her "Julie." Another baby starts crying across the room. Kennedy asks, "Is that one of my babies?" The nursery is one of the strongest and oddest families one will ever encounter. Kennedy stands up. "Thirty minutes until pizza time." I can't believe it. She *likes* the hospital cafeteria pizza. Someday I must get her down the street for an experience with authentic pizza.

Sometimes, a nurse tells me, physicians have a plan but no diagnosis—as with the Blackwell baby. At other times they have a diagnosis but no plan. The latter seems to be the case for Stephanie Christopher.

April 13. Stephanie is shrouded in white gauzes. She is on 50 percent oxygen, 60 percent at night. She is not doing well today. Seems to be slipping. More oxygen is needed to maintain her color. There is more bleeding. Her mother is complaining more and more about how Stephanie is handled. The doctors tend to interpret this as unloading her own guilt on others. But this strikes me as too facile. She may simply be concerned about the comfort of a dying child. Stephanie now gets dusky whenever agitated. She has to be suctioned more frequently. A story is going around that the mother believes one of the doctors is encouraging her to get pregnant again. Randy Hunter scoffs openly at this. There is an interesting question here, though. Since both parents have to have the recessive gene for the child to get the disease, tubal ligation is an issue of some sensitivity. What if the parents get divorced?

Stephanie awakens and is very restless, in spite of the morphine she was given a short time ago. She twists about crying, now slaps at the oxygen mask with her right hand. Both of her legs are wrapped in identical white gauze, a white dress rippled by vaseline ridges. Now she is quiet again. The morphine has probably taken effect.

From the interview with Mr. and Mrs. Christopher.

Mrs. Christopher: There were nurses in there who didn't know anything about what was going on with her—they'd make me nervous. They'd come in there and in order to go in with Stephanie you had to put on a cap, a gown, gloves, and a mask. It was reverse isolation for her, so no germs were going in instead of coming out. And the nurses, boy, they scared me because they didn't know how to handle her. They didn't know how to change her bandages. They weren't sure of what to do with her at all, period. I usually ended up going in with the nurses and showing them how to change her bandages. She laid on a cloth diaper all the time. They had to weigh the diaper before they put it under and, after she'd use it, then they'd weigh it to find out how much she'd gone. The medical stuff with the central line and the G-tube, they knew what to do with that. But as far as taking care of her bandages, there was just no way they knew exactly what to do with her.

Frohock: Would they listen to you when you would talk?

Mrs. Christopher: Oh yes, because I told them. Well, a lot of them knew that I'd gone through it before, and if they didn't, I'd tell them. "I know what I'm doing because I've gone through it before." Because with Katy I'd go in the room and I got so I was changing the bandages and the nurse was helping me, instead of me helping the nurse. I told the nurse at first [with Stephanie] that when she changed the baby, just to come and get me, that I'd be in the parents' lounge. She says "Well, what do you want to do?" I said, "Well, I want to come in and help you change the bandages." She looked at me real funny and she says, "Well, most mothers wouldn't bother going anywhere near the room." I said, "Listen. I have to go back and forth from Allenville [her home town] to Northeastern. I can't take care of her at home and the only way that I can take care of her is while I'm here. Whatever I can do to take care of her, I'm going to do it. If you don't like it, tough, because I want to take care of my baby because I can't do it any place else." She couldn't take a bottle because the nipple would take the skin right off from the inside of her mouth. Neither one of the girls had anything going down through their mouths because it'd just take their skin right off. So I knew pretty much how to take care of them bandage-wise. They'd listen to me because I knew what I was doing.

A small plastic doll in Danielle Raymond's crib is standing in a large bootie. A technician is getting a sonar reading of her brain. He admits that he can't tell from the printout what is happening inside her head. "I don't read these things, you know."

A resident is trying to insert an I.V. into Julia Allen's arm, then her foot, while a nurse sits nearby in a bored (and contemptuous) fashion. Then she alertly stands up when the I.V. goes in—an excitement that is almost sexual. "You got it?" she asks him.

A ventilator starts whining, letting everyone near know that a baby has been removed from her vital oxygen supply. "Put that kid back on the ventilator," a nurse shouts. "I want to hear this song on the radio."

April 14. I was in the nursery both morning and afternoon today. Good conversation all around with staff. They all tell me that Stephanie's mother seems to have a distorted picture of the capacity of the staff to treat her daughter. She keeps telling them, "It's good that now this disease can be treated so much better—that you know so much more now," though no advances in treatment have been made since her other daughter died of the disease two years ago.

April 16. Stephanie is sluggish this morning. She is having trouble opening her left eye. Her head is turned away from the oxygen. Her nostrils are bloody. She is crying intermittently, her mouth open. She appears shrunken to me. Both of her eyes are open now. Her face is contorted from crying. Now she relaxes. She slowly blows a thin bubble of spit from her mouth. The nurse starts suctioning out her throat and trachea with a tube inserted into her mouth. After the suctioning is completed she starts applying what looks like a white sunburn lotion to the baby's skin. Later I find out it is silvadene. The nurse places the vaseline gauzes on top of the lotion. Blisters are everywhere now on Stephanie's skin. Green stool extends from her anus. She is quiet now as the nurse continues to work on her.

Nothing is working for Stephanie. She is still on 75 percent oxygen. The nurses suction her clear every hour. She weighs 1170 grams today. On Sunday her weight was 1120 grams. Hopeful, except that she weighed 1240 grams at birth and reached a high of 1400 grams two weeks ago. She receives .05 mg. of morphine every three hours.

In the afternoon Stephanie is enveloped in fresh white vaseline linens that almost completely cover her body. The nurse is once more suctioning her throat out. Stephanie is more peaceful than she was this morning. The nurse winds up a musical toy. She gently touches Stephanie's forehead. The key in the toy is slowly winding around. I cannot hear the music through the glass window (anymore than I can hear Stephanie cry from where I am standing). The nurse tells me later that Stephanie's oxygen tube is set at 100 percent and she still looks pale and dusky. She could be acidotic. The staff will draw blood gases tonight. She may need another transfusion. She is still receiving hyperalimentation. It has been impossible to feed her any formula.

The nursery is very crowded today. A new arrival late last night was the victim of a comedy (or tragedy) of errors. He was almost a breech baby, a fact not known to the obstetrics staff. The resident panicked and called Susan Markart down from her office (where she was off duty and doing some late-night paper work). Markart managed to deliver the baby and get him into the nursery, though he is at the moment "in terrible shape" (according to one of the nurses). He may be septic. But the treatment now (at last) seems to be appropriate and more successful than the earlier efforts by obstetrics.

A sign on top of Stephanie's bed, placed there this morning by the physical therapist, gives instructions on her care. Then, added to the instructions—in red ink—is the statement "Stephanie likes to be talked to and touched." Touched? The therapist is obviously writing in slogans without awareness of Stephanie's condition. The message continues. "Please try to sooth before giving medicine. She doesn't like wet diapers. Sometimes just a clean diaper, suctioning, and position change will quiet her."

David Quinn, a baby who (like so many others in the nursery) was born prematurely and now, as a result, has severe lung problems and some brain damage, was finally weaned off the respirator yesterday after four months on it. A sign was affixed to his bed: "David Quinn—A star at last!!" with two green stars on it. He was put on an oxygen hood, and his blood gas tests were good with the hood set at 90 percent oxygen levels. But David is back on the respirator today and not doing so well. How transient is stardom.

A nurse is talking about the parents of Cindy Blackwell. "The father must be black. The mother has been here only once and she's white. She was very well dressed, expensive clothes." The Blackwell baby, I notice for the first time, is very dark. "She (the mother) has one other child. Normal. A four-year-old. Likes Michael Jackson." I cannot resist: "And he's normal you say?" The nurse laughs. "But then this one [Cindy] likes Michael Jackson too." A doctor hollers at me from across the room: "Everyone likes Michael Jackson."

April 18. Stephanie's abdomen seems distended again, perhaps because she has no bandages on her torso today. A large red and blue welt marks her rib cage—as if she had been struck a blow (which she hasn't). The thin white tube into her upper chest (through which she is given hyperalimentation) is curled in a loop above her head. The oxygen mask still blows into her face. She is crying, moving restlessly. Her legs and arms are wrapped in vaseline gauze. Some stool, loose and green, is in the diaper beneath her. Her body is slick with sweat and vaseline. This is pure suffering. Is there any point to it? I keep asking myself, If suffering is sensible in order to lead to some good, where is the justification here if all of it leads only to Stephanie's death? A nurse picks her up, lifts her gently over to another bed to clean her linens. Stephanie's eyes are open. Now she is being suctioned. Her color turns slowly dusky.

The nurse repositions the oxygen mask to a point right in front of her face. Stephanie is now quieter, more restful. More "sedate."

Danielle Raymond is smiling, yawning in her sleep. An I.V. is still in her leg, attached to the limb by what looks like a wooden splint. She looks sweet, healthy.

"Moving on Down the Highway" is playing on the radio.

The Blackwell baby is wrapped in thick layers of white clothing. Is she cold? She is sleeping with a ventilator tube squarely in her mouth, one of her fists clenched tightly. She is on top of three pillows with a blanket pulled firmly over her to keep her from falling off the pillows. "Right," a nurse says. "We don't want *her* to wake up." She is back on phenobarbital. More tests are scheduled for tomorrow. There is more talk of sending her to Chicago, where a diaphragmatic pacer can be installed in her chest.

The Quinn baby is enveloped in a flashy warmer—white with spectacular red lining. He is sleeping with the ventilator tube in his nostrils. A nurse is gently stroking his forehead.

4

The resistance of medical staffs to legal regulations and review of therapy decisions has led to the formation of Infant Care Review Committees at a number of hospitals. Northeastern General has had one in place for the last several months. It consists of the heads of the nursing staffs in both pediatrics and neonatology, an attorney, six pediatricians, one lay person, one member of the clergy, and one of the hospital's vice-presidents. The committee is to act as a mediator when parents and physicians disagree on treatment, provide guidance for physicians in difficult cases, and in general function as a forum within which competing parties can communicate with each other and information can be distributed.

I have yet to see the committee notice that is by now supposed to be posted in the nurse's station. But there is much talk today in the nursery about the notice that attendants will not be on duty in the hospital parking garage from midnight to 6:00 A.M. The nurses are complaining about the lack of security for themselves and their cars. There is also a notice of a softball scrimmage on Thursday. Ah! Here it is, framed in white gold, no less, with a covering glass over the printed (not typed) notice. It reads, "Principles of Treatment of Disabled" (from the department of Health and Human Services), and then lists some guidelines—mainly that handicapped infants may not be denied food and "medically beneficial treatment" solely because of their "mental or physical impairments." The list is followed by three toll-free numbers to call if anyone feels that infants are being denied treatment. One is to the physician who heads Northeastern's Infant Care Review Committee, a second is to the state Child Abuse Center, and the third is to the U.S. Department of Health and Human Services. The notice reminds the reader that the "identity of callers will be kept confidential." Or, protection for whistle blowers.

The Infant Care Review Committees can be seen as halfway houses, intermediate institutions between traditional methods of making therapy decisions (leaving them in the hands of physicians and parents) and legal review and regulation. The guidelines are now set by the federal government. After months of negotiation and compromise, the Senate passed a bill (in July of 1984) setting out the principles of infant care that the hospital committees are to implement. Withholding treatment or nourishment under the new law is now a form of child abuse. Failure of a hospital committee to enforce the guiding principles could prompt state legal action. States failing to comply with the regulations can lose anti-child-abuse funds amounting to millions of dollars. The system now in place relies on hospital review committees with legal remedies in the background if the committees do not implement federal principles. It is a system supported (finally) by one of the oddest coalitions in recent political history. Included in the coalition are antiabortion groups, groups representing the disabled, and representatives of the medical professions.

The Infant Care Review Committees are, on the surface, more congenial to the cooperative nature of neonatology than is the legal system acting as a sole adversarial check on hospital practices. The committees combine hospital personnel with community and legal representatives in a discussion forum rather than a tribunal. Though the proposal to have one member of the committee be designated a "special advocate for the infant" was eventually abandoned in the compromise formula passed by the U.S. Congress, there is no reason in principle why the combination of committee review and government check cannot act as an effective arrangement to avoid such tragedies as the Bloomington Baby Doe case. Some health care specialists are offended by what they see as the "Big Brother" attitude of the federal government in therapy decisions. But the head of the review committee at Northeastern is not disturbed by the arrangements. He views the guiding principles as merely a codification of practices the hospital already follows. Nor is he worried about the government as a third party in therapy decisions. "My feeling is that there have been in the past, in some institutions, cases where family and doctors have gotten together and said, 'Let's not do much for this child!'" The hospital committees with government checks will ensure, in his opinion, that a child will receive needed treatment without intrusive government regulations.

Critics of the system, however, predict that the committees will not be used very much. The reason is that disputes over treatment rarely occur among the relevant parties (physicians, parents). Disputes are more often between the relevant parties and the outside world, as in the Keri-Lynn case, where the disagreement was between the physicians and parents, on one side, and the right-to-life attorney on the other. For such a dispute to reach an Infant Care Review Committee someone with access to the case, in the hospital, would have to challenge the therapy decisions or (as with Keri-Lynn) anonymously call in an outside party. This is a rare occurrence. In the first six months that the review committee has been in place at Northeastern, only three cases have been considered. None was a dispute over principles of care; they were all breakdowns in communications between doctors and parents. "Doctors and parents were not talking the same language," the committee chairman said. "Our job (in each case) was to facilitate communication." The absence of disputes over principles of care may suggest that the principles are being carried out in the hospital. But a more likely interpretation is that the system blunts challenges to hospital practices without, except in extreme cases, noticeably changing these practices. No baby will ever again starve to death in a hospital. But the quality of a baby's life is still a factor in therapy decisions without serious challenges.

One might even say that the problems of quality versus life itself are too deep to be handled by changes in procedure. The congressional guidelines for hospital committees identify points at which doctors would not have to begin or continue aggressive therapy. These include circumstances where the infant "is chronically and irreversibly comatose," where the treatment merely prolongs dying or is ineffective in correcting life-threatening illnesses, and where the treatment itself would be inhumane. Any of these three conditions can be interpreted in different ways. The same procedures at different hospitals may lead to different rules for treating infants as interpretations of the guiding principles differ. One asks what would happen if, as cases are decided by review committees, different hospitals develop different practices on infant care. The codification in practice over time raises still another question—whether eventually some hospital committees will begin retrospective and prospective reviews of therapy decisions without waiting for an appeal by an interested party. If such policies develop, and if they are different among hospitals, will parents then be faced with a choice of conservative versus liberal hospitals on the care of their infants?

But the deeper problem is that if reasonable people can give different interpretations to many of the principles guiding infant care, then perhaps the principles do not instruct us precisely enough on how to begin and end treatment. Stephanie's treatment continues day after day. No one is certain any longer about the rightness of this action. The therapy is ineffective in correcting Stephanie's life-threatening illness. It is probably just prolonging her dying. And one could make a very good case that continuing to treat her is inhumane. Yet no one can say—morally, rationally—that enough is enough, for no alternative to what is being done for her makes any better sense. Her doctors and her parents are simply deciding without guidance. There do not appear to be any right answers. Review committees may be good forums in which to talk through the anguish of such choices. Certainly forums seem better than lawcourts for this purpose. But the pain of the choices, and the pain that Stephanie feels, are not touched by more rational procedures in medical decisions.

8
Medical Costs

1

Only one family is known to have paid its own medical expenses in the nursery. Amish parents, who refused all public assistance and insisted on "paying their own way," saved enough money over a two-year period to pay the entire bill for their son's brief stay in the nursery. Most families, however, rely either on private insurance or Medicaid funds to cover their medical expenses. In the absence of insurance or public assistance, very few families in any area of medical treatment could afford to pay their doctor bills. But the distance between private resources and medical costs is particularly great in neonatology. One-third of the families of babies in the nursery are on Medicaid, and the average per-patient costs in the nursery are the second highest in Northeastern General.

The costs of the neonatal nursery are a source of constant concern for the hospital's administrators. The average per-patient per-day cost of a hospital stay at Northeastern is $396. But the variance among units is great. The least expensive therapy is in the adult medical surgery unit at $284 per day; pediatrics is next at $483 per day; neonatology costs $596 per day, with critical care listed as the most expensive at $825 per day. Intensive care (for babies or adults) is the most expensive type of medical therapy and an economic loss for the hospital. Medicaid, the main source of funds for medical expenses in intensive care, pays a maximum of only $341 per patient per day. Anything above that must be absorbed by insurance or private means.

Northeastern's administrators have tried a variety of tactics to control or modify high costs. One of the most controversial is described by one hospital administrator as "going after the physician." Administrators at Northeastern will occasionally write a letter to a physician pointing out that his patients stay longer in the hospital than the average stay, or that he uses more medicine than the average used by physicians. A professional-service review organization in the state (chaired by a physician) regularly looks at the cost records of physicians. Northeastern administrators use these reviews to remind certain physicians of medical costs. To determine standard costs for therapy they also use a complicated formula identifying 23 diagnostic categories and 467 related subcategories, and weighting the categories and subcategories to produce an index of standard costs. These standard costs are communicated to physicians with expensive therapy practices. Administrators also explore with physicians the possibility that a patient's medical problems may be due to a previously existing condition which contributed to the need for a hospital stay. If so, additional insurance and state aid may be justified.

In general, administrators try to solve the problems of costs in two ways: (a) reduce costs by monitoring and then persuading doctors to eliminate unneeded therapies, or by various cost-cutting administrative measures (the hospital eliminated 180 positions two years ago), and (b) increase revenue from insurance and public sources, sometimes through redefining an illness and (often unsuccessfully) by trying to get better rates from the state for Medicaid payments.

Several administrators told me they would like to tell physicians they can spend only x amount of dollars on a patient and no more. But they will not, and cannot, limit resources to a physician who says that a certain therapy is needed for a patient. The reason for their restraint is simple enough. To deny therapy is to make medical decisions, and they are not qualified to make such decisions. The Clinitron bed for Stephanie was illustrative. Several administrators not only told me that the need for the bed was still questionable in their minds, but they asked aloud whether patients like Stephanie should be treated at all. They see enormous expenditures of money for terminal patients as a waste, but do not know how to limit such expenditures. "I can't make these decisions [to limit therapy]," one told me, "but they have to be made."

2

April 19. Late afternoon in the hospital cafeteria. The place is almost empty. Lazy curls of cigarette smoke drift up and away from a nearby table where a doctor is appraising an attractive woman who sits at coffee with him. I am talking to Betsy Randolph, one of the nurses who has spent a lot of time caring for Stephanie.

She tells me about the past, before fear of the law entered medical practice. In the 1950s, she says, doctors regularly administered digoxin to infants who would not survive. This was done in the operating room where the baby could be said to be stillborn. Now, she says, all babies are given a chance to live. At first this was because of a desire to experiment, to see if marginal children could be salvaged. Later, more recently, these medical efforts were constrained by law. Now the dominant attitude is, "Nobody dies on my time," which is translated into doing everything possible to keep infants alive while one is on duty.

Even with this pro-survival attitude, however, doctors will still cut back on therapy when they find that babies are not thriving. Randolph tells me that all babies ought to get maximum support at the beginning. "The Gonzales baby" (a baby in the nursery some months ago), she says, "was premie trash, a piece of protoplasm. But he survived. Right now he's at home. So we have to give the kids a chance." Later, she says, when one is sure that a baby is not going to develop and get better, then therapy ought to be cut back. This is not killing, she insists. It is "fish or cut bait"—give a child the chance to live on his own. "And this is done. There are ways. Steps are taken. Physical care continues but machine care is reduced. Ventilator settings are lowered."

Baby Stephanie, she continues, is a catch-22. There is no machine to turn off. "If there was a machine, and I could, I would have turned it off. Her genes are telling her body that she has no use for her skin. Her death will be one of the most horrible you will ever see. She will have systems failure, a failure of the basic organs of the body when they cannot tolerate any more shock. Then infection will follow and kill her."

After our conversation, I walk back upstairs and go over to Stephanie's room. A new sign is on her window, a kind of Hallmark card: "Please be patient—God isn't finished with me yet." No one knows who put this card up.

April 20. Stephanie is sleeping in a curled up fetal position directly in front of the oxygen mask.

Danielle Raymond is resplendent lying on her back, her hands fluttering lightly. A yellow bootie is on her right foot. She is still under an oxygen hood. She looks eminently comfortable.

David Quinn looks like a small turkey lying on his stomach with his butt up in the air. He is still on a ventilator.

Cindy Blackwell is eerily calm. She seems to be toying with her ventilator tube, her right hand tapping on the metal. She keeps folding her thumbs under her fingers. I am told that this is a bad sign. It suggests brain damage.

Randy Hunter is irritated. A woman twenty-seven weeks along in term is downstairs in obstetrics. She suffers from hypertension. The only successful treatment of hypertension in a pregnant woman is the delivery of the child. The obstetricians took a sonogram and found that the baby is growth-retarded (twenty-three weeks in size) and has hydrocephalus and a variety of other maladies. So, with the consent of the parents, a decision is made to abort with prostaglandins. Unlike other abortifacients (such as a saline solution), prostaglandins induce labor without necessarily harming the fetus. So it is possible that the aborted baby can be "born" alive. And if the baby breathes, the hospital staff is required by law to resuscitate. Here is the source of Hunter's irritation. The obstetricians have defined the medical problem solely in terms of the mother's health, not the life of the baby. They are monitoring the woman only, not the fetus. Yet the neonatologists have been alerted to come down immediately if things go wrong, meaning in this case if the aborted fetus lives instead of dies. So a failure in obstetrics in this instance will be a live instead of a dead baby. And what would normally be a call to help a baby begin life is instead a call to mop up. The obstetrician's exclusive concern for the mother's health may unintentionally produce another patient for the neonatal nursery whose medical problems will be due in part to the therapy administered by the obstetrics staff.

April 23. Stephanie looks—amazingly—better! Is this possible? Only one lesion on her trunk, and it more nearly resembles a large scrape than an open wound. Her thighs are also clear. Her legs and arms are wrapped in a thick white cloth. The rest of her skin looks normal. Her color is good. No—wait—her stomach is a bit rough. But she seems (to me, at least) much improved. She is sleeping well. Kevin Scott, an intern, comes by, however, and tells me that Stephanie's blood platelets are being eaten up more quickly than anticipated. So her appearance is an illusion. She is really worse.

Danielle Raymond is still progressing. She has her ups and downs, her nurse says. Danielle's right foot is wrapped in what looks like a diaper. The nurse tells me that the cloth is there to warm up the baby's blood so that it flows more freely. The nurse unwraps the foot and draws some blood.

Cindy Blackwell is wrapped in a white blanket. Underneath the blanket one can see her pink balloon pants. She is trying to breathe without the ventilator. The doctors gave her a drug last evening that, according to the nurses, agitated her all night.

April 25. Stephanie is on 100 percent oxygen. The oxygen mask is pressed up against her face. She is sleeping at the moment on a regular premie bed while her Clinitron bed is getting serviced. She is still on hyperalimentation. She cannot be fed anything. Everything that is pumped into her stomach immediately passes out through her intestines. The doctors have glumly concluded that there is something wrong with her intestinal tract, though they do not know what. Stephanie is on round-the-clock morphine (every three hours). When the morphine starts to wear off she becomes restless and scrapes her skin off by rubbing her arms against her body. She is, in the nurse's phrase, "slowly disintegrating." No resuscitation is still the standing order "if she decides to leave." I have not seen a physician with Stephanie in a long time. She is currently wrapped (arms, legs) in the vaseline gauzes used as treatment from the first few days of her life.

Danielle Raymond is serene, sleeping on her back still under the oxygen hood.

April 27. Stephanie's vaseline bandages are being changed. She appears sluggish. Her nose and upper lip have been split open by a new lesion. There is blood spotted across the diaper she is lying on.

A new case today illustrates again the ways in which the staff makes decisions on therapy at the beginnings of human life. A child was born this morning with hypoplastic lungs (little or no development of the lungs). The doctors gave him massive support at first. They then examined him in more detail and could not find any kidneys. A sonargram showed only a couple of nubs where the kidneys should have been. A renal scan showed no kidney function at all. The baby weighed 1,000 grams. Dialysis is impossible with a baby this small. The doctors took the parents aside and advised them that their child had no chance for survival. After some discussion the parents and doctors agreed to back off from aggressive therapy and make the child comfortable. The baby had been intubated in the delivery room. The attending physician turned off the ventilator and the baby died. One brief problem was that the baby perked up at first when the ventilator was turned off. But the tests had shown as conclusively as possible that there was no chance for life. The whole event (and entire life of the child) lasted less than twenty-four hours.

The death of the child occurred in room C of the nursery. The room has other babies in it, but was vacated temporarily of nurses not involved with this baby. Only the parents, the nurses on the case, one member of the house staff (Bill Wade), and one of the Fellows (Randy Hunter) were present at the bedside when the baby died. Neither doctor saw any need to call on the Infant Care Review Committee or a hospital administrator.

Hunter saw the decision as routine. "There is no need to involve others who might give erroneous messages to the parents, or create problems. If I had been at all uncertain, then we would have gone in with massive support. But the kid had no chance." Both doctors told the nurses exactly what was going to happen and what the chances were for the baby's survival. One nurse asked about a kidney transplant. Hunter told her that a transplant is impossible with a child so young and in such grave condition. He prepared the parents for the decision by informing them in stages along the way. They were distraught but were able to handle it. The obstetricians were at first optimistic—a common response, according to Hunter, and always unfortunate. But Hunter advised the parents early enough about their child's poor prognosis to avoid coupling their sadness with surprise. Hunter says that "when you bust your butt taking care of a child, you have to make decisions like this. Doctors who do not make these decisions are failing their obligations to their patients."

Again, the viability of the child was the decisive consideration in the therapy decision, and the information was presented to the parents in such a way as to ensure a no-treatment decision—though the parents could have resisted and successfully demanded a continuation of aggressive therapy.

3

From an interview with Danielle Raymond's parents. Mr. and Mrs. Raymond are in their late twenties. Mr. Raymond tells me stories during the interview about hunting and about his wild rides on motorcycles. Mrs. Raymond remains impassive while these stories unfold.

Frohock: Tell me about Danielle from the beginning.

Mrs. Raymond: I don't know what to tell you.

Frohock: Tell me about the birth.

Mrs. Raymond: The nurse and I were the ones that delivered her.

Frohock: How did that happen?

Mrs. Raymond: I was having problems the night before and I talked to my doctor. He told me just to stay home and stay off my feet as much as I could. But the bleeding kept continuing. So he took me in Saturday and told me to stay at the hospital. I was doing fine up until after he left the hospital. Right there I gave birth, right in my room. One of the nurses was with me. She was there. She helped. I did all of the delivering. She just stuck her finger down the baby's throat to get her breathing and she was breathing okay. Then the baby's doctor came in to talk to me.

Frohock: How far along were you at term?

Mrs. Raymond: According to them I was about six months along. I delivered her three months earlier than I was supposed to. I had a miscarriage before I was pregnant with Danielle. Then they came in and told me that they were going to send Danielle to Northeastern General.

Frohock: Did they tell you why?

Mrs. Raymond: Because they said they had better facilities there than my hospital did. My hospital doesn't have what Northeastern General has.

Frohock: Did they tell you what her problems were? (*question to Mr. Raymond*)

Mr. Raymond: No. Well, I didn't find out she had the baby until— she had the baby about 11:30. They called me at 12:00 and told me the baby was dead when it was born. They didn't tell me anything. They told me to call my wife because she was all upset. I called her and she told me the baby was dead. She didn't know if it was alive or not. A few minutes later the hospital called me back and told me the baby was alive. But they asked me what I wanted to do with it. They asked me whether I wanted it to live or just take it off oxygen and let it die. So I decided to see what could happen. I decided to let it live. I wanted to see if it was going to make it on its own or not.

Frohock: How did that question strike you when they asked it?

Mr. Raymond: It felt weird because nobody's ever asked me something like that before. Like they said, "Do you want it?" That's all they said really, and most people would say yes. I did say yes but I didn't know what to say at the time. And then they called me at 3:00 and told me the baby was getting ready to be shipped out. Then they called me back at 5:00. During all this I didn't have a car. My car broke down and I was staying with my sister at the time because she lived closer to the city. And we got out and her car broke down just as we got there. So neither of us had a car to get in. It was snowing pretty bad that night, so I couldn't hitchhike into the city. I wouldn't be seen when I was hitchhiking. So they kept calling me and letting me know, and that was about it.

Frohock: Did you have the feeling if you said *no* to the question that they would have just done nothing?

Mr. Raymond: Probably. Because at the time . . . Well, this last time I went out to the hospital the doctor came in and he started reading off the thing—I guess a dictaphone or something, so he could have it all transcribed for her records—and he said something about her being fourteen minutes without oxygen before she was resuscitated. So they must have waited quite a while before they even called me or anything.

The decision to resuscitate Danielle Raymond, in short, was made by Mr. Raymond on the phone without a moment's notice. No time to reflect, to think through the decision—he was asked what he felt should be done and, on the spot, made a decision. Mrs. Raymond was not consulted at all.

Frohock: When she was born, did the doctors or the staff consult you on whether to resuscitate the baby?

Mrs. Raymond: No. They had to rush me into O.R. right away because I was bleeding too much. As a matter of fact, the doctor went ahead and said it's a wonder I pulled through because I lost so much blood. He didn't think I would make it because I was white as a ghost. They were concerned about me, too. Then, right before I went into O.R., they wheeled me over to the maternity ward where all the babies are and let me see the baby—they were planning to take her to Northeastern. Then when I got of O.R. and went to recovery, the nurse came over and asked me if I wanted to see the baby before they sent her to Northeastern. And they brought her—the ambulance was there waiting—and they brought the baby over to me before I went up to my room.

Frohock: You saw her then a second time?

Mrs. Raymond: Yes.

Frohock: How did she look to you?

Mrs. Raymond: She looked good. She looked like she was going to pull through. It was kind of scary to see her like that. She had on one of those little hats and was in oxygen and all. The nurse that was with her gave me a booklet and all and told me what hospital she was going to be in. She said if I had any questions and if I felt up to it, to call the hospital.

Mr. Raymond was more shaken by the appearance of Danielle in those early days. He could not bring himself to visit her after he saw her the first time—not until she grew and began to look more like a normal baby.

Mr. Raymond: I never got to see her until I went to Northeastern. Then when I did see her—well, I went into the room where they had her and I could see her heart beating right through the skin. She was real skinny and I could see the bones just about. And right then I decided, I can't come back down because she doesn't look like she's going to make it. I see her right now and I don't want to see her if she gets worse. I used to take my wife and my mother down, because they used to always go down and visit the baby, and I'd wait in the waiting room. I wouldn't even go into the special area. I'd wait over on the other side. Then once I decided to go back in and see her and I started going back down all the time. She'd gotten better since the first time I'd seen her. She looked like a real baby then. The first time I saw her, she didn't even look like a human to me. She was all brown and had a lot of hair on her and it just scared me in the beginning.

Danielle Raymond's problems continued for days and weeks. At one point (as we know) she almost died and was brought back by the physicians and nurses at Northeastern General. Mr. Raymond described this event to me as he saw it when it occurred on March 21.

Frohock: Did you ever at any point along the way—did they ever make a call like that again to ask you if they should continue treatment or simply stop trying to save her?

Mr. Raymond: No. Well, they called up once, but I wasn't here. I was out helping a friend pull some logs out of the woods. There was something wrong—I don't know what—but when I got home everybody was at Northeastern. That sort of had me worried because she still wasn't doing good and there was a chance that—they told us right there the first time we went down, it was within seventy-two hours whether or not she would make it. Well then they just kept adding that seventy-two hours every time we went down. It was still chancy all the time. When I got home, nobody was here and a friend of my mother's came over and told me what happened—that something happened to the baby and they wanted the parents there right off. I called down there right when I came back in the house and found what was going on. She was just having a little bit of a problem but they didn't know what was going to happen at the time.

Frohock: Did they tell you what those problems were?

Mr. Raymond: Mainly her heart. She wouldn't breathe. There wasn't any breathing and they also were concerned about her heart. They thought maybe they were going to have to do the heart surgery there. So a friend of my mother took me down to go talk to the doctor. I wanted to be there to find out more myself what was going on because they couldn't really tell me more on the phone.

Frohock: And when you went down there that time . . .?

Mr. Raymond: I talked to her doctor and he said they had everything under control. They went ahead and decided to start giving her a kind of medicine that closes the valve up in the heart. This was in the afternoon. By the time we got down there, everything—she seemed to be doing all right.

The staff at Northeastern saw the Raymond parents as indifferent about Danielle. Mr. and Mrs. Raymond have different views. They explained their absences from the nursery in terms of "doctor's orders."

Mrs. Raymond: I wanted to go up and stay at the Ronald McDonald House the first couple of weeks, but the doctor thought it best if I stayed here for a while. Because if I got too close, he was afraid something would happen.

Mr. Raymond: He was afraid if she got too close to the baby at the time and something did happen, it'd be to much for her. So he figured it was best that we went down every once in a while for a visit instead of staying down there.

I asked Mr. Raymond in some detail about his decision to resuscitate his daughter—why he made the decision, what his thoughts were at the time.

Frohock: When you think back on the decisions—did you come close to saying *no*?

Mr. Raymond: I wasn't quite sure what to say at the time. I didn't know what the baby looked like. I didn't know what was wrong with her or anything at the time. They didn't tell me anything. They just asked me whether or not I wanted to keep her and I figured—well, I was in a bad car accident four years ago and I died four times. I figured I made it, she might. So, give her a chance to make it on her own. I shouldn't make that decision for her. It's up to her. If she's going to make it, she's going to make it. If she's not, she's not. It's going to have to be up to her mostly. So I guess she was a fighter.

Frohock: Do you feel in looking back over the treatment that your daughter got that the doctors provided you with enough information along the way?

Mr. Raymond: The doctors in Northeastern provided me with all the information I wanted. They told me everything that was happening. They told me what would happen if something did happen to her, what they'd have to do. They had me sign some papers so in case something did happen and we weren't there at the time, they could take care of it right then. Plus they had me sign some other stuff, experimental drugs or something they were using—they had me sign for them. I figured that they know what they're doing, so they wouldn't be giving it to her if it wasn't going to make her better. I signed whatever they wanted to just to make sure she was going to make it.

Frohock: On decisions of the sort that you participated in, on life and death, resuscitate or not to resuscitate, do you think on the whole that parents ought to make these decisions? Or doctors? Or some combination? Or what?

Mr. Raymond: I figure the doctor should have made it. If he had thought that something was going to be wrong with her or something, or if she wasn't really going to make it, then he should have made the decision instead of calling me and having me make the decision. If I had made the decision and something happened to her then it might have made me feel worse. But he should have made the decision, then called me if she had died or something. Then I wouldn't have known she was really born or anything. I would have thought she was born dead or something like that. It would have made me feel just as bad. But I think it would have made me feel worse if I had made the decision and then she had died or something, or something worse had happened to her.

Mr. Raymond told me at the end of the interview that he calls Danielle the million-dollar baby. The Raymonds live in a very modest house next to an elementary school. To someone of their means, indeed to anyone of any means, Danielle's medical bills must seem to be nearing the threshold of a large fortune.

4

Medical costs are increasing generally in the United States, and neonatology costs are no exception. One of the special ironies of neonatal medicine is that increased costs are in part a consequence of medical success. Infant mortality has been steadily declining in the west for over two centuries. The explanations for this decline are widely accepted: People in affluent western societies live better than they did in earlier historical periods. Good nutrition is possible both because of improved food supplies and better information (widely disseminated) on adequate diets. Housing has improved. Water is cleaner and safer. People are healthier as a result, including babies. The development of immunizations against a wide range of diseases and the use of antibiotics to combat bacterial infections have further decreased infant mortality. Prenatal and postnatal medical care is superior now to any treatment in the past. It may be that toxic wastes and nuclear disasters will reverse these encouraging improvements in health prospects. But in high-income countries infant death rates have declined, and continue to decline substantially. (The 1981 rates were half what they were twenty years earlier, for example.)

As infant death rates decline, medical technology plays an ever larger role in the reductions. The skills exercised in neonatal nurseries contribute to improved survival rates for premature infants, infants with severe infections, and those with the range of birth defects now commonly encountered and treated by neonatologists. The cost of such contributions, however, is increased by the very fact of declining infant death rates. The marginal cost of each success in saving a life can be expected to rise as the death rate continues to fall; for the infants who continue to need treatment are those who have not responded to two centuries of improving health care and thus are the most recalcitrant cases. Further, the probabilities of successful treatment may also decline as the death rate falls, and for the same reason—the most difficult cases will be those last to respond to treatment.

How much does neonatal medicine cost? Estimates vary, but no estimate places the cost below other, less-intensive medical therapies. The Blue Cross Association, understandably concerned to estimate medical costs with some precision, has used three types of costs to calculate neonatal care. One is infant direct costs (those assigned directly to the patient); the second is unit direct costs (those assigned to the level of neonatal care—intensive, intermediate, and growth and recovery); and the third is hospital overhead (those costs allocated to all three levels of neonatal care). The infant direct costs include nursing and physician care (the latter from itemized bills), supplies, ancillary tests, and services provided to the infants. Unit direct costs include depreciation of facilities and equipment (based on percentage use) and nonmedical staff salaries. Hospital overhead covers building costs (on the basis of square footage in use), administrative and data processing, even laundry and linen. A 1982 study using these three categories calculated the average cost for infants (using a sample of ten babies) at $312 per day. Infant direct costs amounted to 51 percent, unit direct costs 23 percent, and overhead 26 percent of the total. Nursing care accounted for 24.1 percent of the total costs (or almost half of infant direct costs).

The figure of $312 per day is below the figure cited by Northeastern's administrators for the neonatal nursery ($396 per day). But taking both figures together suggests roughly the per-diem range for infant intensive care. The aggregate costs for hospital treatment very greatly among infants (depending upon how long they must remain in the hospital). Four of the ten infants in the Blue Cross sample survived. Six died in the hospital. The total cost of care for the survivors ranged from $14,659 to $40,752 (over stages ranging from sixty-two to one hundred days). Among the six infants who died, only one lived more than four hours. The bill for this longer-term survivor (nine days of life in the hospital) was $7,594. The five babies who died quickly had bills ranging from nothing to $505. Other studies show a similarly wide variance in total costs for intensive infant care. In a study of a hospital in California, total bills from July 1976 through the end of 1978 averaged $8,069. In nineteen out of the 1,185 admissions tallied, however, the cost was in the $50,000–$99,000 range. Five infants had bills of more than $100,000. These costs, as might be expected, reach impressive totals when summed for the entire country. One estimate (reported in 1978) for the total annual cost of neonatal intensive care in the United States is $1.5 billion. (These latter figures are cited in Strong, "The Tiniest Newborns"—see Bibliography, section 3.)

In the nursery at Northeastern, there is almost no discussion of health costs. Concern in expressed from time to time, mainly in the form of worry about how skyrocketing costs are to be brought under control. Most of the worries are expressed by hospital administrators, who are caught between a medical emphasis on the best treatment for each individual patient and the hospital's need to balance revenues and expenditures. The medical staff at Northeastern may limit treatment on a judgment that a baby will not benefit from therapy. But they never consider limiting treatment because it is too expensive.

5

April 28. A family is in the hall talking to Bill Wade. The father looks like a tired version of Ronald Coleman—he has suffered too many defeats. The mother-in-law looks to be domineering. The mother is putting one aggressive question after another to Wade with her husband and mother-in-law as audience. Wade seems to be holding his own.

Stephanie was given oxygen manually last night. She had bradycardia (slow heart rate) and was revived with 100 percent oxygen applied to her face. She also received blood this morning and looks very pink right now. There is a large abrasion on her left cheek. It is covered with a bandage. A nurse at the desk tells me she has some real questions about the oxygen—whether it should have been given at all.

There is more activity in the nursery today than during the last few days. A fetus (doctor's description) was born this morning at 600 grams, 25½ weeks. No resuscitation was needed, so no decision was required. The survival rate for a baby this small is less than 20 percent. The staff is giving him all the basic therapies: warmth, keeping him dry, oxygen if hypoxic, fluids with sugar through an I.V. It is on infants like this that the staff divides over treatment. Catherine Richmond ventilates all babies like this one. Paul Montgomery procrastinates though he gives the appearance of making decisions. Susan Markart and Bill Wade (without worrying about appearances) will look at a baby for some hours, and then—if the infant has, say, a heart rate of 30, is uttering agonal gasps even with an oxygen mask near his face, seems in general to be making no effort to survive—they let the baby die. If, however, the baby makes an effort—has a higher heart rate, is breathing on his own, moving around, wriggling—then they go all out to save the baby. The baby born this morning, Robert Beak, did get his heart rate up to 140 and is breathing. So *now*, if he takes a turn for the worse, every member of the staff is prepared to make all efforts to resuscitate. Clouding this baby's prospects is the fact that he is not moving much. His blood gases are good, however, suggesting that he is breathing well. His beginnings were auspicious enough. While the doctors from the nursery were working on him in the delivery room, a nurse "completely lost it—flipped out." She returned to the nursery and announced to everyone that "the baby is dead."

A second set of arrivals this morning also is presenting interesting problems for the staff. Twins, delivered at twenty-eight weeks. The obstetrician delivered the first one without incident. Then he had trouble getting the second one out. The nurse in attendance describes the scene as "a disaster." The twin's arm was sticking out though the obstetrician kept fumbling around (as if he couldn't find the baby) "for an eternity." Since blood is diverted away from the baby by the mother's body as soon as an incision is made, there was a long oxygen and blood deficit while these efforts were being made. The nurse reports that "I just kept watching his [the baby's] arm and it kept getting blacker and blacker." Finally a delivery was made. At the moment this second twin is doing very poorly, though his brother is doing (understandably) better. Each weighs slightly over 1,000 grams, so there is no issue of not resuscitating.

I walk over to Robert Beak's crib. He is a long and very thin infant. His weight, according to the doctor standing with me, is generous for his gestational time, but it is stretched out (he is a *very* long baby) and so doesn't help him as much as it would in a shorter baby. He is on CPAP. A technical problem is facing the doctors. The baby's trachea seems too small to accommodate the smallest intubation tube made (2.5 cm.). So the staff cannot intubate him without doing great harm to his trachea. No one knows at the moment how to solve this problem.

One of the interns describes to me the strangeness of the delivery room downstairs in obstetrics. There, five to six people (the group brought there if any trouble is expected) are periodically gathered between the legs of a woman. The room, according to the intern, is very cold. The intern (as do many others in the nursery) ridicules the views of obstetricians. Usually, he says, they are over optimistic about a baby's prospects, misleading the parents into expecting too much from the neonatologists. Sometimes, though, they are pessimistic in opting too quickly for an abortion. He also says that obstetrics is riddled with paradoxes. They will call the neonatologists down for problems in 25–26-week deliveries, yet they sometimes abort 27–28 week fetuses.

It is evening. A large red blotch extends down Stephanie's left cheek, which is split open near the jaw line. She now has a vaseline gauze on the side of her head. Her entire body, arms and legs included, is completely covered in white gauze. A large cotton swab is under each arm. She is sleeping with her face six inches from the oxygen mask. A new pink teddy bear is on her bed.

April 30. Robert Beak is under a cellophane wrap covering the top of his bed to keep him consistently and uniformly warm. A warming lamp is shining light directly on his body—he is in the spotlight. White eye patches held on by a wrap-around bandage protect his eyes from the light. A white stocking cap is on his head to keep his skull warm. He is restless, his long arms hitting up against the cellophane wrap as he sporadically and weakly flails about. A nurse remeasures with a tape Robert's distance from the lamp. There are the usual heart-lung monitors on his chest and thigh. He was

intubated this morning successfully by a physician who somehow inserted the 2.5 cm. tube into his trachea without damage.
The nurses describe the feat as "awesome" in its level of skill.
"Threading a needle when the thread is bigger than the opening"
one tells me.

The weaker twin is getting worse every hour. The staff are afraid
that he has level 2 scarring of his retina. Problem: Since high levels of
oxygen *or* carbon dioxide correlate with retinal problems, then how
should his lungs be treated? A double bind exists. Almost any
treatment of such a newborn will have undesirable consequences on
his vision.

6

Ignorance as well as skill is the source of composition fallacies in
medicine. Several doctors have shared with me their worries over
the outcomes of treatment. No one knows with any reasonable
certainty the effects on children of some of the things done in the
nursery. One doctor tells me that they are in the 5 percent range of
predictions—that doctors are unconditionally right in their prognosis in only five cases out of every hundred. This low level trans-
lates into a mandate to *treat*. If one has so little certainty on measures
designed to maintain life, one must give the infant all possible
chances to survive. The other consideration is success. Neonatologists save many more infants now than they did even a decade ago.
A higher proportion of children in neonatal nurseries also survive
intact. But one byproduct of improved skills is that a larger number
of children are also living at the margins of human existence, damaged beyond repair.

The problem of marginal children will probably always be a
byproduct of producing more intact children. To see this, one needs
only alter the percentages. Suppose certainty of prognosis could be
raised to 99 percent, so that one would be wrong about the outcomes of therapy in only 1 percent of all cases in the nursery. The
issue of whether to treat all types of maladies in the 99 percent zone
would still exist. But even if that issue were resolved—a ranking of
quality-of-life conditions successfully set and measured against life
itself in early therapy decisions—the problem of treating marginal
children would still occur, since the 1 percent uncertainty would
lead to severely damaged infants.

The high value we ascribe to life itself is the source of our commitment to treatment when uncertain about outcomes. Most doctors

would treat a child even if there were 10,000–1 odds against survival. Stephanie Christopher is being treated in the face of odds even greater than that. The possibility of marginal survival does not compromise this commitment. Suppose that out of a set of five infants, treatment leads to the survival of two—one intact and one at a marginal level of life—and to the death of three. Now suppose that a medical improvement would lead to the survival of all five—three intact but two (or twice as many as before) at a marginal level. Is the improvement worth it? Of course. Life is too valuable to be abandoned just to avoid marginal byproducts. This is roughly what has occurred in neonatology in the past decade. Further improvements will refine and tailor therapies to specific syndromes and blunt the adverse side effects of treatment. But only perfect certainty (unattainable in medicine, perhaps in life itself) would eliminate the Jill Monihans produced by medical treatment. Nor is there any foreseeable therapy for such children. Medicine cannot in any conceivable future reconstruct neurological functions. It follows that even if most areas of ignorance are changed into areas of knowledge, medical therapy will still produce damaged survivors condemned to live a marginal existence.

Cost constraints may finally limit the extended treatment of such survivors, and perhaps even neonatal therapy in general. But such constraints are hard to justify on moral grounds. There is first the old problem of value incommensurability. Some items do not fit on a common scale. In *Sophie's Choice*, Sophie is told by a Nazi commandant to choose which of her two children is to be sent to a concentration camp, and which one is to accompany her to what she thinks is survival. She cannot choose. The commandant responds that he will then send both children to the camp. In desperation she decides to send away the younger child, a daughter, and to save the older boy. The choice finally drives her to a despair close to death. The economist who says that under duress Sophie assigned different utilities to her children is on a different level of despair, worse off than Sophie even in her agonies. Some things cannot be compared and ranked, a limitation that critics of utilitarianism have pointed out for more than a century.

Assigning a price tag to life seems to be a case of combining incommensurate values. Jack Benny's stock gag (never failing to get a laugh) was the long, contemplative pause following the mugger's threat, "Your money or your life." Part of the amusement is due to the absurdity of the pause—of course your life is worth more than your money. But another part is surely due to the craziness of Benny in trying to compare life and money. The denial of Stephanie's Clinitron bed met with strong opposition from the medical staff at Northeastern. The cost was minuscule, they said, when compared to expenditures in the nursery. But this misses the point. Suppose the bed's cost had been prohibitive. Would high cost have justified the denial? The point is that we have no scale to provide common weights for cost and life. Each consideration—cost, life—is located in a different community of values. Cost considerations derive from the marketplace, where goods are commodities to be bought and sold. The values placed on life are drawn from religious and philosophical traditions hostile to market values. To place a price on moral items is to denigrate them, to undermine their status as goods independent of monetary considerations.

The moral justification of cost limitations is even more difficult to make when scarcity is examined in medical practice. Scarcity in medical resources is not a physical limitation on available goods. It is a social decision reflecting society's priorities. The costs of maintaining even current levels of medical care are considered very high by many hospital administrators. But high according to what standards? Most estimates of the annual cost of neonatal nurseries in the United States fall in the range of $1.5 to $3 billion. Even on the higher figure, neonatal expenditures are dwarfed by the total expenditure for health care in the United States of more than $160 billion per year. The figure of $3 billion amounts to roughly 0.05 percent of the U.S. national budget. Defense allocations annually cost more than eighty-seven times what is spent on neonatal nurseries. It is also important to remember that medical care at the beginning of life pays more dividends in extending life than at any other time. The physicians in the nursery at Northeastern are aware of these long-term benefits. They point out that a child who survives intact can live seventy to eighty years. If dollar costs are somehow assigned to human life in opposition to moral traditions denying such an assignment, the benefits to society of such a long life can amount to considerably more than the costs of treatment. In the Blue Cross study, it was pointed out that the four infants in the sample were saved at an average cost of $26,000 apiece. When compared to a widely cited social value assigned to an adult life—$200,000 to $600,000—the neonatal intensive care figure is only a fraction of the social benefits successful therapy can provide.

Cost thresholds can be reached where even rights to medical care are overridden. Rights trump utilities—but not where the thresholds of social need are high and the benefits of rights are unintelligible. One hidden variable in all calculations of neonatal costs is the expense of follow-up or extended treatment. Such treatment has a dark side. All survivors of neonatal nurseries do not end up on the benefit side of the ledger. Many infants live with such severe defects that they are liabilities to all concerned, including themselves and their families. The costs of such continued support (for example to Jill Monihan) have not been accurately calculated. But in cases where extended treatment is all cost and no benefit, the Blue Cross projection of long-range returns is meaningless and the proposition that such infants have a right to further treatment does not make much sense.

Society provides a number of strategies to resolve conflicts between communities of value. The oldest, prominent in classical Greece, is to obliterate one of the communities. The logic is impeccable in homogeneous societies. If exclusive principles define values in public life, the political society cannot tolerate the existence of diametrically opposed values. One set of values or the other must give way for the political community to sustain itself. Doctors in the nursery did tell me that they half-believe that the hospital administrators would like to eliminate the nursery entirely, a Carthaginian proposal that administrators respond to with amused silence. But it is unlikely that the extreme Greek response to alien communities would be seriously pursued in neonatology. If it did, its logic would extend to all crisis medicine and even to technological innovation itself in medicine. Like the librarian happy when the library has all of its books *in* rather than checked out, a hospital with a balanced budget and no important medical care would make no sense in terms of the purposes of medical practice.

The modern pluralistic solution to community conflict unfortunately makes as little sense as the draconian measures of ancient Greece. Market and medical values might flourish together in a stable cost structure. But the tolerance of mutual accommodation is difficult to conceive as medical costs continue to rise. Every doctor and administrator interviewed, and all empirical indicators, anticipate greater not lesser conflict between costs and therapy. In the sense in which scarcity is always with us and reflects a social allocation of priority goods, nothing is new in this conflict. But medicine's increasing reliance on technological innovations leads most respondents to the belief that some special, perhaps unique confrontation is coming that will force society to make comparisons between values that philosophers view as incommensurate. Nor does it seem possible to respondents that society can conceal these comparisons in the way, say, that the actual costs to human life of the automobile in contemporary life are obscured. Most individuals interviewed believe that the choices will be both forced and open.

Speculation is natural on how these choices will be framed and made. Obviously some hard choices will have to be made among equally viable candidates for therapy. Theories of distributive justice routinely affirm the natural pluralism of selection criteria—need, desert, merit, for example—and the absence of any satisfactory device to rank the criteria. Should society select its best or its most needy for life-saving therapy, for example? No answer can persuade everyone, even philosophers. Perhaps an Aristotelian model of friendship will help. Imagine how a community of friends would settle on the allocation of scarce primary goods. Certainly the neonatal nursery, especially in the most critical times, is more like a community of close friends than a collection of strangers. But the imaginative exercise can also conjure up the divisive affects of hard choices on friendship. It may be for this reason that a lottery is often used, even between lovers, to settle on those choices which are unthinkable as cold, rational decisions.

If cost considerations are to limit any type of treatment, however, the limitations must be settled at some aggregate level as an issue in social policy. The staffs at neonatal nurseries cannot introduce such restrictions. No doctor or nurse I interviewed was prepared to say where and how expenditures should be reduced (though most said that some limit has to be imposed). Physicians make therapy decisions on the premise that the patient should get the best treatment available. Medical staffs are constrained by this logic to be partisans for medical expenditures. Physicians do not profess to be authorities on economic issues or impartial judges of whether society is spending too much or too little on medical care. No one treating a patient like Stephanie Christopher will or can say that treatment must be limited because enough money has been spent on this case. Not even hospital administrators are easy with such decisions. If cost is to limit medical treatment, the interviews suggest that the limitations will have to be settled at some distant remove from medical practice itself. Society, in one of its decision-making institutions, must determine economic limits to medical expenditures and, in doing so, settle its own priorities among primary goods.

9
Medical Practice

The real neonatal nursery is not at all like most television renditions of hospitals. Most of the activity is routine, even tedious. Sometimes neonatology reminds one of the description of an airline pilot's job as thousands of hours of boredom punctuated by a few moments of sheer terror. Life-threatening events in the nursery, of course, occur more frequently than airline emergencies, but when they occur there is still no sense of drama. The staff kids around to stay relaxed and effective.

The nursery does constitute a community. There are four primary groups of individuals: doctors, nurses, patients, and families. Other players are found in the nursery but they have bit parts. The key to understanding the nursery community lies in the fluid and complex relations among these four primary groups. Three patterns are particularly intriguing. One is the relationship between patients and the three other groups. One might think the patients would be passive receptacles for the emotions and attitudes of others. That would be a mistake. The patients, though without the ability to speak or even think in any developed way, exert strong effects on those around them. Michael Anthony is a decisive figure in both the professional and private lives of Mary Jane Kennedy. Stephanie Christopher has deeply affected all who have come into contact with her (including me). The infants, moreover, have inchoate personalities. They resist or accept treatment, respond to or reject affection— and such actions place them in a network of human emotions in the nursery. Nurses, for example, do bond with some infants and not others, and doctors regard some infants as attractive figures and others not. The families of the babies form connections with their progeny, not with other babies. But even here the variations are substantial. Some parents are deeply committed to their children, others abandon them. The capacity of the babies to be endearing, to seem "human" and responsive, is an important ingredient in whether parents connect strongly with their babies. In complicated ways the infants are decisive figures in determining communal relations in the nursery.

A second pattern is found in the relations between staff and the families of the babies in the nursery. Both nurses and doctors talk to families. Nurses are the primary contacts for families. They provide information and comfort. In most cases they try to walk a thin line between the pain that a full and objective disclosure often brings to parents and the soothing effects that a gloss would have on parental worries. The nurses are good at negotiating this balance. They get involved with families. Some families they can't abide, others they love. In general, however, they seem able to present the child's medical problems honestly, yet expressed with an intimacy that seems to soften the bite of even the most tragic situations. The parents generally see the nurses as tough and amiable characters whom one definitely wants around when events get tight.

The relations between doctors and families are more complicated. Parents, as expected, have favorites among the doctors. The favoritism does not seem to turn on professional expertise but on congeniality and accessibility. A doctor who is too professional, too "clinical," is not well regarded by families, even if highly respected by colleagues. The doctors, in turn, evaluate parents in terms of (a) an ability to comprehend medical information, and (b) a commitment to their children—in that order. An articulate and intelligent parent always gets high marks from doctors. Unfortunately this kind of parent is as unusual in the nursery as in any other area of life. Because of the awe with which most families view doctors, the relation of parents to doctors tends to be unequal. The physician is authoritative.

Nowhere is the inequality between parents and doctors more clearly expressed than in the transmission of information. Most of the time physicians will fairly and lucidly lay out various options so that parents can make a choice. But when they want parents to select a particular option, they will present the facts of the case and the proposed therapy in terms designed to sway the parents. For example, by labeling a therapy as "experimental" or "untested" or "new and radical," a doctor can be reasonably sure of a negative response. If the negative choice is still not forthcoming, the doctor can say that the therapy is "unknown" or "of marginal benefit" of has "unpredictable side effects." On the other hand, if a doctor describes a therapy as "promising" or "improved" or "hopeful" or "quite possibly effective," the parents are more likely to select that treatment. Over 50 percent of the parents of babies born with hypoplastic left heart in Northeastern General reject bypass surgery for their children. The doctors describe the surgery as "experimental" and say that "no one will be mad at you if you don't choose this surgery for your child."

The physicians are not fooling the parents with such guidance. The language they use to set up options expresses their best medical judgments on the condition of the child and the advisability of therapy. The mortality rates for hypoplastic left heart approach 100 percent whatever the treatment selected. But it is a mistake to think that parents are the equal partners of doctors in assessing their children's condition and choosing therapy. The paradox is that the more rational and receptive a parent is, the more likely he or she is to accept the doctor's perspective on the child's care. Doctors will share more information with parents who can absorb and comprehend it. But sharing generally means accepting the doctor's point of view. The less rational and understanding the parent, the greater the distance between parent and doctor. A greater distance can lead to parental independence in choosing therapies. When parents are influenced by community values far removed from, and even antagonistic to, the guiding principles of medicine, parents and doctors may disagree sharply. Jill Monihan's mother believes in miracles, a divine intervention that doctors on the whole do not subscribe to. Using religious resources, Mrs. Monihan has been able to block all medical efforts to end treatment of her badly damaged child. An adamant parent can force treatment of even the most hopeless cases (including trisomy 13 and 18). The more irrational and uncomprehending a parent is on medical standards of reasoning, the greater are the chances that the parent's child will be treated when the benefits are marginal.

A third pattern marks the relations between doctors and nurses. Many doctor-versus-nurse clichés seem borne out in neonatal care. The nurses are more affectionate, more nurturing of the patients, than are the doctors. They treat and care for the whole patient while doctors tend to treat diseases rather than persons. Doctors are the recognized specialists on medical matters in the nursery. The nurses admit to this, but they claim to be the authorities on the needs of the baby they are tending. When doctor and nurse disagree on treatment, the nurse will argue for what she thinks is best for the child. But the end result is always the same. The doctor's views are implemented, not the nurse's. Nurses rank doctors according to their skills in treating patients. They speak with contempt about the abilities of some physicians in the nursery, and praise others to the skies. The savvy doctors always try to get the nurses committed to a course of treatment. In the informal give-and-take of the nursery, life can be miserable for a doctor the nurses think incompetent or just plain wrong. But in a crunch, the doctor prevails, for the doctor is authoritative on medicine; the nurse, finally, is a subordinate.

This hierarchical pattern was illustrated dramatically by an event that occurred in early May. David Quinn had been getting steadily worse since his brief moment of freedom from the respirator. His breathing problems in particular had been slowly multiplying. One morning, while Rebecca Smith was routinely tending him, he suddenly stopped breathing and his heart stopped beating. Smith reacted swiftly: "Get the doctors in here—now," she called to a nearby nurse. The nurse snapped a button on the intercom system found in every room and announced the emergency. Within seconds, doctors were around David's bed. One doctor immediately began pulmonary-heart manual resuscitation. Another—Bill Camisa—reintubated him. (His intubation tube had been removed earlier in the morning by doctors to allow the nurses to suction his trachea and pound his back to clear the phlegm out of his bronchial tubes.) Another doctor injected a stimulant into the baby's body. Still a fourth began an I.V. in his scalp. David's breathing and heartbeat were restored within a minute. "Welcome back to the living," Camisa told him. Then, to the assemblage, he announced that, for David, "It's back to base one now on his treatment."

At a later moment in the resuscitation efforts, Camisa peered into David's throat with a magnifying instrument and determined that the intubation tube was not in properly. "Okay, David", he told the baby, "you're not going to like this." Then he removed the recently inserted tube and replaced it with another. After Camisa was satisfied that the tube was in and the respirator was breathing again for David, the group broke up to give the X-ray technician a chance to take a film of the baby's lungs and check the tube placement.

After David had been stabilized there were words between one of the doctors, Jay O'Brien, and Rebecca Smith. O'Brien, arriving at David's bed after the baby had been brought through the emergency, proceeded to antagonize all the nurses at the bedside with the pronouncement that carbon dioxide levels in a baby's blood are not relevant indicators of the baby's need for ventilator support. Since Smith had warned the doctors earlier that David's high carbon dioxide levels and normal pH factor (degree of acidity or alkalinity of the blood) suggested that he should be put back on the ventilator, she naturally felt both vindicated by the baby's arrest and angry that he had almost been lost. In the altercation with O'Brien she invoked her "seven years' clinical experience" in defending her views. "I will also use what happened to this child as evidence for what I'm saying." O'Brien responded with the doctor's synoptic eye: "One case does not make a scientific theory."

After the two separated, Smith was furious. "I have never heard a bigger crock of shit in my life," she announced to everyone within earshot. O'Brien told me later that the "danger in this [Smith's] view is that the nurses will tell David's parents that someone is to blame for what happened here."

Later I talked at length with Smith about her experiences with doctors and in the nursery in general.

> *From an interview with Rebecca Smith. Smith is young, bright, engaging. She knows her craft and herself.*

Frohock: Tell me about what happened to David Quinn.

Smith: It was very frustrating because they allowed David to sit all Sunday night with high carbon dioxide levels. That can be just as toxic as low oxygen, and they let him sit like that. They made a conscious decision Sunday night not to do anything, to wait until they got the blood results Monday morning and if it was still bad, then they would do something about it. And I went to do his care at 8:30, and you know how wild he is. He was literally flaccid, blue, not moving any air. Diane was in charge. She was walking through and I said, "Diane, get me a doctor." The doctors were on rounds and they said put him back on his CPAP. I said "Fine, but I want somebody in here." So Dr. Camisa came in, listened to him and ordered bronchisol aerosol treatment, which will open up the airways. They use it for asthmatics. And while the respiratory fellows were setting up the CPAP and the Bronkosol treatment, he arrested. Within thirty seconds he just quit breathing and his heart rate went down to zip and that was it. They just pushed him too far and that was all right except Jay O'Brien walked in afterwards and said "CO_2's of 100 are fine. You can wean a child on that as long as his pH is compensating." I said "You've got to be kidding! Look at this kid. You going to tell me that you could leave this kid with a CO_2 that high for that long and he tolerates it? I don't think a respiratory arrest is particularly tolerating it." He said, "Well you can't base your judgment on one child," and I said, "I'm not. I'm basing it on seven years in this place." And I'm still mad at him. I have no respect for him. That was the stupidest thing to say.

Frohock: Do the nurses and doctors often disagree on treatment?

Smith: I was talking with Betsy afterwards and she said, "You know, probably if you've worked here as long as you have, you see trends." One thing that was particularly amusing to me was that five years ago you never put respiratory babies on their abdomen because it supposedly increased their carbon dioxide level. Then Dr. Richmond read a study and so we started putting every single respiratory kid on their abdomen because they thought it decreased the carbon dioxide levels. One week we were doing one thing and the next week we flip-flopped and did the exact opposite because somebody read a study. You see these things and—it depends on who's on and what their philosophy is. It changes from month to month depending on the doctor, and your standards of treatment change depending on who read what study.

For the past seven years it's been obvious to me and the kids—never minding what somebody's study with poor control shows—that the kids don't tolerate carbon dioxides of 100. And this so-called doctor, who I have no respect for anyhow, comes in and tells me that he can tolerate it when I just got through with a respiratory arrest from a kid who obviously couldn't. I really was feeling a little hostile at the time. I had all I could not to rip him up and down personally, which I didn't do and would love to have done. It just depends on what study somebody's read and the kids suffer because of it. Because somebody's hot on some new study they read about.

Frohock: And the nurses are basing their judgments on their clinical experience with the kids?

Smith: Yes. We don't have the technical background that the doctors do and I know that. I know when I'm qualified to make a judgment and I know when I'm not. Now, I might not know all the ins and outs of the respiratory impairment that David Quinn has. I don't know the depth of what the doctors know. But I know how a kid like that reacts. I know when he looks bad. I know when more intervention is needed. I know when a kid's been pushed to the point where you can't push him anymore. I know the babies.

In the interview Smith stressed the importance of looking at the child instead of just the numbers on the test returns. She ranks doctors by how well they are able to read the child's condition holistically, by looking at everything and sensing the whole baby and his problems.

Smith: Your good doctors, the doctors that you feel take good care of the patients, are the doctors who will come in and look at the patient clinically. We had a baby one time that was in—I couldn't tell you the name. I couldn't tell you exactly what was wrong with the baby, but she had terrible fluid and electrolyte imbalances. We were having a horrible time keeping all the numbers right and making sure she was hydrated. We didn't know when she was hydrated and when she wasn't hydrated. Susan Markart came in and looked at the kid, I think she was a resident at the time, and she said "My God, this kid is so dry." The baby's fontanel was sunken in the head. I mean it was just—and that's a sign of dehydration. Here they had this kid so screwed up because nobody had a handle on where the kid was. They were just looking at numbers. They couldn't figure the numbers out and nobody but Susan came in to look at the baby and see what the baby looked like. They get so tied up in their numbers and their treatments.

With David Quinn this morning they were talking about trying to wean him down on the amount of respiratory support we were giving him and trying to wean him off the aminophylline drip, which is a continuous medication drip. Mary Wood [an intern] was the only one who said, "I don't think David will tolerate doing both those things at the same time." Two doctors who I don't think are that good were talking about doing both things at the same time. The one doctor who I thought was good, who's the one who comes in and looks at the kids, says, "He's not going to tolerate that." The doctor who will come in and look at your baby and look at your child clinically instead of just your numbers, is your better doctor. Your nurses will look at both numbers and patient, and that's why I think sometimes you have to stop the doctors and say, "Wait a minute, come look at this kid."

This tension between nurses and doctors over treatment is typical of what I observed. Doctors are more theoretical, nurses more oriented to what they see as the practical needs of the babies—though some of the doctors also seem to have that special insight that allows them to see the whole patient that the nurses care for on a daily basis.

Later in the interview I asked Smith what she thought would happen to David Quinn.

Smith: My guess is that David will never go home. If David goes home, he might stay home for a month and come back in the hospital for a couple more months and die.

Frohock: Should these babies be treated at all in the first place?

Smith: That's the ultimate question. I guess what I've learned is I'm glad I'm not in the position where I have to make that decision. I've learned that I'm damned happy I'm a nurse and not a doctor. I don't want that kind of responsibility. And a baby like David is a shame. But there are a number of kids who were David's size who did perfectly fine and are great little kids. I think, yes, you have to treat them because you don't know if they're going to turn out all right or not. That's the scary part. If you had the foresight to know who was going to live and not be maladjusted in some way, developmentally or whatever, that'd be great. But we don't have that. And there are some kids who die who never should have died. There are some kids who should die, who never die. And sometimes there's no rhyme or reason to why a kid makes it or doesn't make it. So that's a long way of not answering the question.

Frohock: Let me make it even harder. Once we do know, much later on, who's going to make it and who's not, should we then stop treating those who are not going to make it?

Smith: Could you take David's oxygen away?

Frohock: No.

Smith: Neither could I. If there was a more acute, critical baby who would die in a matter of hours, one hour, turning off a ventilator when you knew that the baby had mush for brains, I could do it. But I can't do it to a baby like David, who you know would suffer terribly over a period of quite a bit of time. I couldn't do it. I couldn't take David's oxygen away. I think it would be a terribly cruel thing. I think, in David's case, it would be murder. In another case where it's a more acute baby, a younger baby, a baby that there's no question is going to be damaged and it's a very simple matter of turning the pressure down on the ventilator or something like that, to me, somehow in my mind, that's not quite as murderous.

2

May 2. Stephanie was not breathing this morning when the nurse checked her. The nurse immediately raised the oxygen level to 100 percent and started suctioning to clear her trachea. When these efforts did not affect her breathing, a doctor injected her with narcan, a drug used to counter the effects of morphine. Five minutes after the injection she began breathing on her own. The staff is puzzled over what caused Stephanie's respiratory problem. Her heart rate was a steady 40 beats per minute thrughout the ordeal, which is unusual. When babies "crash" (sink rapidly), a doctor tells me, they have irregular heart beats—40, then 60, then 40, etc. Also, Stephanie's main line goes into her heart. So if the accumulated morphine was the cause of her arrest, then the heart rate should have been affected along with the respiratory distress.

Stephanie is also now on antibiotics again since one of her blood cultures grew—and quickly this time (three days rather than five). She looks terrible: restless, soaked in vaseline from her gauzes, lesions all over her body. Her respiratory rate is 80 per minute now, though it was at 120 per minute after the injection of narcan. The nurse caring for her tells me, "She must have said, 'This is my death for the week.'"

I have a bad cold today, so I stay in the halls and make the visit short to avoid infecting the babies with the virus that is currently abusing my body. Later in the afternoon I call to see how Stephanie is. The nurse says, "Stable. She hasn't pulled any more stunts." I ask her about Stephanie's prospects. "Not good. She is not going anywhere. No weight gain. Nothing."

Do not underestimate the physician's impulse to treat no matter what. Bill Camisa was the attending physician who administered narcan to Stephanie this morning. He also began the antibiotics. Later in the afternoon he wondered aloud whether this had been the chance to end her agony. He could have delayed the antibiotics and narcan by insisting on additional tests, or he simply could have refused treatment until Stephanie was beyond help. But he did not, could not, seriously consider those alternatives when he was faced with the decision. He simply treated the patient. So there really is a switch now to turn off to stop Stephanie's ordeal and Camisa had his hand on it. He simply couldn't bring himself to turn it. Camisa also had some words for those who would discourage treatment of children with short-gut problems (and who live only a few years in the hospital on hyperalimentation). Just look in the eyes of those children, he said. You have to treat them.

May 3. A public address announcement in the nursery tells of a postmortem beginning at 1:00 P.M. for Harvey Luce (whoever that is). The nurses begin telling of the autopsies they have attended. One says, "I was okay until they cut open the head." Another: "Me, too. Same thing. Mine was a tall fifteen-year-old who had died of leukemia. He was so tall he took up all of the table." Still another: "We had to go to at least one autopsy in nursing school." The first nurse: "We did, too."

Stephanie is restless. Her bottle of hyperal and its connecting tube is hung over her shoulder. A large jar of white cream is open on her bed. (A tag is on the jar: Stephanie's). She is a greasy figure twisting on a bed. The oxygen mask (as always now) is near her face.

One of the twins died this morning—the one the obstetrician had not been able to find at first. A nurse tells me that everyone in the room was crying when the baby died. The father was devastated. He kept saying, "It isn't fair." He and his wife had just bought a bigger home to have room for the twins. At times like these I can see how very human such events are, and how each of these babies is a member of some larger community, where death means something other than it does in the nursery. For the doctors, death is a loss, a failure. The adversary of life has won. For the family of the child, death is a grievous personal loss. Both groups are concerned for the child. But the family attaches a unique value to their child that the doctor cannot share. The different attachments to the child are represented in different styles of acting in times of stress. Doctors will make jokes during emergencies to avoid stress and tightness. No parent selects this style. For them stress becomes oppression, weighing on them like the heaviest blanket in the world. It is no wonder that the two groups—the two communities represented by families and doctors—are kept separate during emergencies. Only after the doctors' efforts have failed and the child is irretrievably dying (and the items of medical care viewed as grisly by the families, including all monitors, tubes, etc., have been removed) are the parents allowed into the room to hold the child. At these moments the community of family attachments dominates. The family, the attending physician, and the nurse assigned to the child attend to the rituals of death and grieving. This different setting can then affect everyone, family and staff, in deep emotional ways.

Robert Beak, the thin and premature baby, is struggling. Camisa says, "Beak is doing poor to mediocre for a baby, great for a fetus. So it depends on your point of view."

May 4. Stephanie is being plastered by the nurses with a white cream. The gauzes are placed on top of her skin. Her color is better today, though there are more lesions on her face. The attending physician tells me that this morning they bandaged Stephanie's arm and she then proceeded to scrape the bandage across her face and open up her forehead and cheeks. So she is now sleeping with major scrapes across her face, self-inflicted. The physician says that "that's an unconquerable situation in there" (Stephanie's room).

A baby who has graduated from the nursery successfully (he is not going upstairs to pediatrics) is being transported home. The baby is in an incubator on a luggage sled alongside two large suitcases. The mother is in a coat standing near the sled. An ambulance attendant asks the nurse what the baby's first name is. "Giovanni," she answers. "No, I mean his first name." "Giovanni," the nurse repeats. The other attendant reads the mother's surname off a chart and asks the mother what her maiden name is. "That is my maiden name," she replies. She looks at him in a nice moment of silence. "Oh. Where do you live?" he continues.

A baby with chicken pox is in isolation. A nurse is in attendance inside the baby's room. I ask how a baby catches chicken pox in a neonatal nursery. No one knows.

Danielle Raymond is crying silently under two layers of glass— her oxygen hood and a glass sheath that covers her bed. She is wearing real baby's clothes for the first time, a blue nightgown with several bows on it. The glass isolette being used on Danielle is designed to maintain the air temperature around her close to a normal body temperature (98.6°F). Premature babies have trouble maintaining body temperatures. They have a lot of skin surface proportionate to their body weight and so they lose heat more rapidly than full-term babies. Their skin is also thinner than that of full-term babies, and they have less fat in their bodies to produce heat. The alternative to the isolette is an open bed with a heater placed on top of it. (This is the system currently used to keep Robert Beak warm.) The problem with an open bed is that room breezes will alter the temperature (which is why Beak's crib is currently enveloped in cellophane). On the other hand, every time the door of an isolette is opened, the temperature inside changes. The open bed has one other advantage over the isolette. It allows the staff to get at the babies quickly in an emergency. So acutely ill babies are kept in open beds with warmers. The chronics and those acute babies who have passed some critical threshold (as Danielle Raymond has) are kept in isolettes.

A new sign has been posted on the wall in room A from a recent graduate who went home: "Thank you—Love always, Matthew Bogner." The message on the card appears under three balloon pillows held by a clown.

May 5. Bill Camisa tells me that we need an artificial placenta (not a womb—this would be too ambitious, I suppose). Some device that, like a heart-bypass machine, would allow the lungs of premies to develop while the child is living on the machine without using his lungs. He said that something like this is in fact around. But it doesn't work so well. The babies die on it.

Death is something everyone on the staff wants to avoid for their patients. One intern describes the mentality as "No one, but I mean no one, is going to die on my shift." The competition to cheat death is fierce. If a patient dies, the interns on duty feel they have somehow failed, even if the death was unavoidable. Those not involved think, "Not while I'm on duty."

I recall a scene in a bad movie I saw as a child (I can't remember the title, but it starred Frank Sinatra and Robert Mitchum) where a senior physician tells a young doctor to listen to his old heart with a stethoscope. The young doctor gasps at the sounds he hears in the old man's chest. The old doctor smiles with dignity. Today the old man would be jerked onto a heart-lung machine. Life is different. Movies can't be made like that anymore.

May 7. Stephanie is sleeping restlessly on her left side, arms in front of her face cradling the oxygen mask. There are dressings on her head, torso, legs, arms. A white cotton ball has been placed directly below her rectum. The nurses say she is about the same.

Many "pit-stop" babies were admitted last night. These are babies who are ill but are on the whole healthy. No one expects them to stay very long in the nursery. Several new premies are also on the floor. The staff had to send one eleven-day-old case upstairs to pediatrics. No room in this inn today.

In the afternoon, in the midst of this newly charged pace, a photographer arrives with a hospital public relations woman and an elegantly dressed elderly man from hospital administration. Publicity photographs are to be taken of a wooden rocking chair donated by the family of a patient who recovered. A nurse is found to sit in the chair holding a wrapped-up doll (a simulated baby) and a bottle of Similac complete with nipple. She is positioned near one of the beds. The photographer takes the picture. Thanks all around.

Hospitals are human communities, and are themselves broken up into smaller communities of specialized forms of care. In all the units there are friendships, levels of professional expertise, consumers, producers, lovers, strong emotions embedded in the expected competition, and conflict among able professionals. The staff in the nursery is obsessed with competence, with doing their work at a high level and not damaging the patients. This concern over quality makes failure much more painful and success the sweetest of highs.

From the interview with Rebecca Smith.

Frohock: What's the worst thing you've seen here, Rebecca, since you've been here?

Smith: The worst. I don't know if I can give you the worst. Let me think. I think some of the worst things I've seen have involved poor doctoring. There was this vaginal breech delivery that I went to that I will never do again. And I remember one of our chronics, in the middle of the night, extubated himself. I remember spending four hours holding that baby and restraining that baby while somebody tried to cram a garden hose down his throat, and the only reason it took four hours was because it was an incompetent doctor. In the morning at 8:00 a good doctor came in, pulled the tube out, and put one down the baby's nose lickety-split, and I spent four hours helping to torture that baby.

I've seen some gross and disgusting kids but they'd die, thank heavens. I think the worst things I've seen have been things that we've done to babies. Stephanie. We had a baby in C nursery a couple years ago, Crying Don. Ask some of the nurses about him who have been here. He was—I don't know how old he was when he finally died. I was never involved with him. I took care of him two or three times. But some of the girls were highly involved with him and he was a case of pure and simple torture. That baby had—every bone in his body was broken. He had a central line in. He had a colostomy. He had heart defects. He had everything wrong with him and he was in agony. He was on a ventilator and it was just pure agony. To take care of him was so hard because you knew the poor kid just needed to die. No one would want to live in the kind of pain that he lived in for months.

To me those are the kind of things that are the worst. The things that we do to them. We had a baby here five to six years ago. All the doctors know her because she's still seen over at the State Hospital for dialysis. She was a little premie, not too small and wasn't doing well. They took her for a heart catheterization and didn't find anything. Then a week later they took her back, found a major heart defect, and did some minor heart surgery on her. They put in a high umbilical venous line, which clotted off both her kidneys, and they had to take her into the operating room. They put in a catheter in her abdomen so they could dialyze her. They call it peritoneal dialysis, which is a temporary form of dialysis. People long-term get regular blood dialysis. And they thought for a long time that she would get her kidney function back. We just did everything we could to kill that baby and she didn't die. She had so many holes in her abdomen that when you put the dialyzing fluid in it would spurt out the holes. We used to call her the Williams Memorial fountain. I mean we did everything we could. The child got an overdose of morphine, ten times the normal dose of morphine, and we had no way to dialyze her to get rid of the morphine. For three weeks, we had to give her narcan, which is the medication you give to counteract narcotics. She's, I don't know, six or seven years old. She's got the developmental capacities of a two-year-old. She's a little charm, but, you know, "Here's what you've got, Mrs. Williams. Take your kid home." She lays in the bed in the dialysis unit over at the state hospital with her feet up by her ears. She just likes to lay that way. Weird kid. "Here, here, we saved your daughter. Take her home."

Those are the worst things. The kids that we just did everything in our power to screw up. We had a baby—I can think of another one. She was a little premie and she had a horrible seizure disorder, and they finally decided we should let her die. So we put her in an isolette in B nursery. When she had her seizures, she'd go out for four minutes. Her heart rate would be 40. She'd be blacker than the ace of spades. We weren't allowed to touch her because she was going to die during these seizures. She's at Touchstone Developmental Center. She never died. She's still kicking around. She's six years old or something like that, I don't know. You think that kid would die? Never. That's why Stephanie's not going to die for two more months. The kids who are supposed to die, don't.

Frohock: Have you ever had kids that just die who aren't supposed to?

Smith: Oh, yes. That's sad and that's devastating. It happens. Babies who are supposed to do fine but something happens and they don't make it. Those are usually kids that . . . There's beta strep. That is just so devastating. Its supposed to be a big beautiful baby and they come in with this cherry-red glow. I can pick one out like that. The doctors can't do it. We had a kid a year ago that came in, was real sick. I said "It's strep." They said, "No, he's pink. It can't be strep." I said, "It's strep." Two days later, cultures came back. It was strep. The kid died because they didn't start antibiotics. Why should they listen to a stupid nurse like me? I mean, they started them, but not for ten hours or twelve hours or something and you can't do that. When you've got a strep, you better hit them first thing with antibiotics. Those kind of kids are sad. And there are kids who die who aren't supposed to. But for some reason, they don't stick in my mind as much as the ones who won't die. They just keep hanging on.

Frohock: Well, what's the best thing you've seen since you've been here?

Smith: Best thing? We were talking about this today at lunch. We haven't had one here. PFC baby? We haven't had one . . .

Frohock: Persistent fetal circulation?

Smith: They're one of the sickest kids we get. I mean they are awful and unless you can break the cycle that goes on in PFC, unless you can stop that cycle, because one thing worsens the other and the other thing worsens that and they just keep hitting each other up, the kid just gets worse and worse and worse. Unless you can stop it, they'll die. And I remember a nurse, who doesn't work here anymore, sat and worked with that baby the whole shift. Every chance she had, she vibrated this kid's lungs. For some reason it opened his lungs up. Now, you can't say—I mean who knows? Maybe the kid would have opened up had someone else taken care of him and not done that. You never can say for certain—well, it was definitely this or definitely that—but she worked with that kid and that kid opened up and did great, no problem, went home. That's the kind of thing that's the best. That kid should have stayed in the cycle he was in for three or four more days and maybe died. But those kind of things are great too. I don't know if I can give you a worst or a best. I don't know if there is a worst or best.

I know a best. We had—I can't think of her name. She was back in G nursery. I can always remember the room they were in. Diana could tell you her name. I'll think of it in a minute. But she was another baby who was a skin baby like Stephanie, but not the same disorder. By looking at her, you'd think similar. She also had no bone in her skull. She just had like a membrane over her head. You could actually see the gyri of the brain through the skin. And she had all these open lesions. They initially put her on antibiotics. I think she got two or maybe three doses. Then they called Children's in Boston to see what they ought to do with this kid. They said just d.c. [discontinue] the antibiotics, put saline solution dressings on her, and leave her alone, and she'll die. She didn't die. The doctors never went in her room. It took us four months or something of reverse isolation, nothing but nursing care. We'd go in and spend an hour with her and feed her, take her dressings off for the hour and let them air out and dry, and then you'd start it all over again. She healed all her skin and she grew bone in her head. There are certain kinds of cells that can either go into tissue or bone. I think they're mass cells or something. She went home, and she eventually grew the bone.

And this was a kid that they left to die, who was never supposed to make it. Never had enough antibiotics. The doctors were never in her room. They didn't do a hell of a lot for her. It was all nursing care and she went home and did great and she's a happy little kid. That's one of the best things. She was great. I wish I could think of her name. We had a sign up over her door. G was her room and it's a sign that she was the original cuddle bug. And she was. She would love it. When her three hours of isolation were up and you'd go back there and feed her, she'd play and laugh and giggle with you and look at you and she was the cutest little kid. I remember we got a picture of her a couple of years later. It's one of my favorite pictures. She's sitting on a beach in a regular lawn chair, wrapped up in a big striped, real bright striped towel with a little hat on eating a popsicle. She was just the cutest little kid and the nurses were so proud. We were all so proud because we did it. And she did it.

3

The pediatric unit at Northeastern is where the babies go who do not fully recover in the neonatal nursery. It has thirty beds, eighteen of these located at a side of the unit devoted to less intensive medical care. There is a large activities room in the middle of the floor near the nurse's station. It is filled with toy building blocks, books, tables, and has a large movable screen that can separate activities. The atmosphere is less hectic than in the nursery. The children up here are beyond the point when they need constant and intensive medical treatment. But the mood of the staff is more solemn. The patients here sometimes represent the worst and most intractable problems in pediatric medicine. The nurse in charge, Nancy Todd, tells me matter-of-factly, "We treat what they send us."

Two of the most frequently mentioned children in the nursery are Jill Monihan and Joey Graham. Jill is the baby whom the staff continues to treat because her mother is adamant that treatment continue. She is lying inert on a normal-sized bed in a semiprivate room. Jill is now twenty-six months old. An I.V. tube extends from her left arm. The respirator makes the only sound in the room. It is startling to see a child of this size with a breathing tube extending from her nose and mouth to a machine. A nurse is quietly changing Jill's pillow case.

Nancy Todd is in a reflective mood as we leave Jill's room. "Sometimes we trick ourselves into thinking that we don't die. Everyone is going to die. Some die young, some die old. In the meantime I give the patient the best care. And that's all you can do."

Joey Graham celebrates his second birthday next week. He is what the staff calls a short-gut child. He was a premie born with a portion of his intestines outside his body. For some reason the birth occurred in the obstetrician's office. The doctor, who was a country doctor and inexperienced, "totally freaked out," in the words of the nurses. Joey was transported to the nursery at Northeastern, but by the time he arrived a lot of his intestines had died. The surgeons at Northeastern removed the dead bowel and saved as much of his intestines as they could. Since he was not a standard necrotizing enterocolitis baby, the staff was optimistic that he would recover well enough to feed normally. But apparently he lost some vital sections of his intestines and never did well. He has been on hyperalimentation for virtually all his life and cannot tolerate any formulas. No one expects him to live much longer.

At this moment he is standing next to a table in the activities room, a central line attached to his body and extending to the ever-present hyperal solution suspended from a mobile metal stand. He is an attractive child with delicate and fair features. His hair is blond and combed neatly back from his forehead. He is playing at blocks with a nurse. He looks at me briefly as I stand in the doorway staring down at this alert child. I am told that everyone falls in love with him. I can see why.

As I walk away down the hall, I see a sight that will always be with me. A two-year-old girl is sitting up in her crib with tears streaming silently down her cheeks. Her mother, in a wheelchair, has just left. The feeling of emotional isolation felt by that little girl is so sharp it is palpable, like a sharp breeze one feels on suddenly turning a corner away from shelter. She cannot talk. She wheezes questions to the nurse trying professionally to comfort her. The nurse tells me in an aside that the little girl's name is Laurie Masters and that she suffers from spina bifida and a variety of other ailments. Laurie gives and receives strong emotions. She loves her mother very much. Is this a life? Yes—though with more pain than most of us ever see. Laurie's life is lived behind the bars of her crib. Her only constant companion is the roommate in the bed next to her, another patient who is so young and sick that he cannot speak. I try to imagine days and nights for Laurie Masters. Hospital routines for feeding and bathing. Footsteps in the hall. Nurses checking her vital functions (as they say). A parade of visitors during certain hours of the day. The quiet darkness of a hospital at night. Loneliness. That is Laurie's home, and her world.

Later I ask Peggy Ryan, the head nurse in the neonatal nursery, what a no-code instruction permits and denies. She tells me no CPR (cardiopulmonary resuscitation). No bagging (oxygen). Usually yes on antibiotics. But no use of bicarbonates, epinephren, calcium gluconate, atropine, dextrose. A no-code instruction would lead to

Jill Monihan's death (in all likelihood). But no-code issues do not bear at all on the lives of Joey Graham and Laurie Masters.

From the interview with Rebecca Smith

Frohock: What do you do to unwind? This is a high-stress environment, it seems to me. Very demanding.

Smith: You just forget it. I allow myself, when I go home, to think about what's happened. I get in the car, I turn the radio on and I drive, and I'll go over what happened during the day. Then when I get to the babysitter's, that's it. I shut it off. I might think about it while I'm cooking dinner or something. But when it's family time, I don't think about work. Because you could let it consume you if you wanted to. I was thinking about David Quinn last night and sometimes, like Monday, after David's arrest, I am hyped all day. I went home and told my husband about David, which I don't usually do. But I knew I needed to tell him about it. If I told him about it and he knew what happened, I could drop it. And I did. I think I said "God, I feel bad for David" or "Boy, it pissed me off." But shortly thereafter I'm able to drop the subject and forget it.

I think later that night I did call to see how David was doing. But I didn't discuss it with my husband again because he doesn't want to hear about it. He can't tolerate hearing about sick kids. So, if it was really wild and it's still driving me crazy, I'll tell him about it to get it out of my system. But then it's got to be dropped. It's the same thing if you had a fight with your husband the night before and you come in in the morning and you're still upset. You get involved in what you're doing at work and within an hour you've forgotten about it. I do the same thing at home. I might be hyped up, but I get involved in my home life and you forget about it, you turn it off. You have to.

But you see, that's why I'm a nurse and not a doctor. When you're a doctor, you can't do that. You don't have a home life, and I'm not willing to do that. My husband says, "Why don't you go to medical school?" I'm saying, "Are you crazy?" I don't want to give up that much of my life to work. It's not that important to me. The money isn't that important to me. He says, "You could make so much money." I say, "I don't care. I've got a life to live. There are things I want to do." So when I'm at work, it's work, and when I'm home, it's home. As much as you can isolate it, I do. A lot of the girls come in on their days off for staff meetings. They go to baby showers and they go out to happy hour together after work. I don't do that. When I get out of here at 3:00, I'm home and that's where I want to be, with my daughter, with my husband. I don't want to be with the people at work. I work with them eight hours a day. I'm not interested.

A social practice has purposes and rules. The nursery has no formal, defining rules such as the rules that define games of chess or baseball. There are instead summary or practice rules developed to achieve medical goals. The Hippocratic oath is a pledge to do no harm and to preserve life. The activities of the neonatal nursery are organized to achieve these purposes.

Unfortunately the two main purposes of medicine—health, life—can conflict with one another. It is not always clear what the physician's responsibility is when this conflict occurs, for the deep moral principles of medicine lead to contradictory imperatives. Hyaline membrane disease, for example, requires artificial respiration in most instances. To keep some infants alive, ventilator settings must be fixed so high as to destroy lungs. Harm is done by preserving life. The contradictions of neonatal medicine are even broader when patients like Jill Monihan are considered. There is virtually no possibility that Jill's health will be restored. One can even argue that she has never been in a state of health in her twenty-six months of life. The doctors are simply trying to keep her alive. Whether the practice of medicine ought to be organized to maintain life at the expense of health is the central issue in neonatology today.

10
Communal Rites

1

May 9. Stephanie's mother is in the room with her. Mrs. Christopher is fully garbed in sterile white, stroking Stephanie's forehead lightly. She leans over to a point a few inches from Stephanie's face and begins talking to her softly. Stephanie is awake. Her eyes are open and she appears to be listening to her mother's words.

Obstetrics has acted in an unusual way. Tomorrow they are delivering a baby whose presence in the mother's womb has been a threat to the mother's health and life. The standard treatment in such cases is immediate delivery of the baby, which, given the gestational time, would be an abortion. But the woman wants the child. So the obstetrics staff delayed the birth a week to push the baby over a twenty-five-week threshold, even with the risk this delay posed for the woman.

Danielle Raymond has improved so much that she has been transported to the local hospital in her hometown. There her parents can visit her more frequently. She no longer needs the intensive care facilities at Northeastern. Looks like a happy ending. Danielle was dressed in a white nightie with blue spots when she was transported, and appeared to be a normal, attractive baby.

The nursery is very active today. Many new babies are here from obstetrics and more are on the way. I walk over to Stephanie's room. The nurse tells me that she is "the same, the same, the same." Everyone seems resigned to the fact that she will never get better. The mood around Stephanie's bed is now more like a death watch than the attentiveness of a medical care facility. I dreamed all of last night about Stephanie—that she was moved to a different location, that different treatments were being tried on her. I wonder if the nurses and doctors dream about their patients.

The practices of the neonatal nursery do not favor authoritative, rational decisions. Many agonizing choices do not have to be made. Events dictate conclusions. (Patients die, or recover, in ways that mandate therapy decisions.) When decisions are required, they are often the result of protracted discussions, negotiations, even bargaining between parents and doctors. Even in these broad discussions a number of predecision conditions affect outcomes. The patient (again) can worsen or improve dramatically. The parents' educational levels and general receptivity to the physicians, the physicians' choice of language to describe the child's condition and the prospective therapies—these elements clearly affect the decision to treat or not to treat. Even the history of the staff's experiences bear on therapy decisions. If, for example, the nursery has recently treated and failed to save a baby with necrotizing enterocolitis, an "Oh, no, not again" reaction is common when a new NEC baby appears. Staff resistance to another baby Stephanie right now is very strong. The doctors and nurses would try harder at this point to convince parents that treating epidermolysis bullosa even at the beginning leads only to heartbreak—which it has for everyone connected with Stephanie.

These predecision conditions diminish the role of rational decisions in the nursery, and they strongly affect therapy decisions when such decisions have to be made in hard cases. The case of Ryan Flynn illustrates many of these features of neonatal decisions. It is instructive to pay close attention to the way this baby is received and treated, and how his physical condition eventually comes to dominate the staff's responses to him and to his parents.

The case starts on May 9 with a call for a transport from an outlying hospital. The child has "multiple anomalies," according to Bill Camisa (who receives the call), and the local doctor "pushed the panic button" and had to be talked through an examination of the baby. The nurses who will transport the baby leave in the hospital helicopter.

An hour later the nurses call in. They have reached the outlying hospital and have just examined the child. Their report intrigues everyone who hears it. Ryan Flynn has no kneecaps or elbows. He has hydrocephalus. Small lungs appear on the X-ray. Camisa tells the nurses to give the baby ampicillin; they will get more blood cultures here at the nursery. The baby is on the way. The nurses at Northeastern prepare a crib and move some equipment over to the bed. The irreverent comments begin. "When is the Gila monster arriving?" a nurse asks. Everyone reacts with disbelief when they hear for the first time that the baby has no knees or elbows. Randy Hunter observes that "you can't play second base in that condition." A nurse responds: "You can *be* second base, though." The part that disturbs the doctors most of all, however, is that the baby was intubated in the operating room when little information was available. "It was a monumental decision," Hunter says.

At 5:00 P.M. the baby arrives. He is brought into the nursery in an incubator by two uniformed pilots and is accompanied by the two nurses who transported him. The doctors immediately examine Ryan. They think his left leg is broken at the hip. His sexuality is anomalous. He is a big baby. The scales show him at 1330 grams. His eyes are half open throughout the examination. Ritiglia runs his hands over Ryan's back. "I detect scoliosis." Ryan was a breech baby, delivered by cesarian section. His Apgar score was 1–3. Camisa reads aloud the family history. There are many bony irregularities in the family: missing vertebrae, missing ribs, extra bones. The important question to Camisa and Ritiglia is not the bone condition per se but whether there is a syndrome present which will present other neurological problems. Since Ryan is currently being oxygenated manually (bagging), a decision has to be made on whether to attach him to a ventilator. Here the doctors are cautious. They have examined the baby visually and manually. An order for X-rays in the nursery has been sent down to radiology. But the staff wants to avoid committing a ventilator to the baby until they know more. The problem is that the doctors need a CAT scan of Ryan's head to get the information they need, and bagging cannot be continued during the scan. Do you ventilate for the CAT scan and then remove the ventilator? Everyone is skeptical about this option, fearing the legal implications. Hunter suggests an option that is adopted—a CPAP for two quick CAT cuts of the head.

Joe Ritiglia sits down at the nurse's station as Ryan is wheeled out to radiology. "My instincts tell me to do nothing with this kid. But bone abnormalities can be consistent with a breech position. And bones can heal and those babies can go ahead and lead a relatively normal life. I need more information.

Bill Wade has joined the examining team. "You have three abnormalities here. And one of them is possibly no brain." He describes how he has just shined a light on the front of Ryan's head and the whole upper region lit up like a pumpkin at Halloween. A normal brain would make the area opaque. Instead, it is translucent. "You also may have no or little lungs. That would give you your out." He means justification for not treating. The third abnormality is of course the anomalies in Ryan's bone structure.

A nurse comes over and tells Wade that Ryan's head circumference is 40 centimeters. Wade tells me that 36 to 37 centimeters is the upper limit for a full-term baby.

One of the nurses who was part of the transport team says that the doctor at the first hospital thought initially that there was not enough amniotic fluid. It looked as if Ryan was pressed to the side of his mother's womb. But when they cut into the mother there was too much fluid. "It splashed all over the floor," one of the nurses said. "They had to wipe it up with a towel."

The results of the CAT scan on Ryan are brought to the nursery shortly after 6:00 P.M.. They show that there is brain substance. The translucence experiment was false. Also, the unusual size of the head is due to bone, not swelling (which is unusual). There is some expansion of the lungs. Ryan's left leg is broken, as the doctors suspected. The doctors—Ritiglia, Hunter, Wade—agree that now they must give Ryan the benefit of the doubt and continue with treatment.

"Get blood gases and bag the kid with 100 percent oxygen," Ritiglia tells a nurse. "Then call the parents." He says he will tell them that their son's condition is consistent with, but not diagnostic of, a bad brain.

The nurse on the transport team reports that the parents were not surprised or shocked by Ryan's bony abnormalities. "We expected that," they told the nurse. They were concerned only that their baby live.

Hunter is pessimistic about Ryan's prospects. "I'd bet Ritiglia's future wages that this kid will not turn out normal neurologically. But we don't have enough hard data to do anything but support him."

Ritiglia agrees. "I can't pull the plug. I'll support him."

A nurse asks if they can get an EEG tonight.

Hunter replies that it would be difficult. "But even if we could, it would not help us in making a decision." He explains that children who have a hard birth can have an abnormal EEG for a while and turn out all right later.

Another nurse comes over. "I move the leg that's broken and he doesn't do anything. There's something wrong. Now he's starting to smack his lips."

The group of doctors goes over to Ryan's crib. Hunter looks in the baby's eyes. An intern strolls over. "A little nativity scene," he comments. The nurse is still bagging Ryan. Hunter takes blood from the baby to check his blood gas levels after ten minutes of 100 percent oxygen. Ryan's pupils do not react to stimuli. He does not respond to pain in his broken leg. Nor to the needle inserted to draw blood. There is some speculation that he may be paralyzed.

The nurse leaves with the blood sample for the laboratory. Four minutes later the gas report is brought in by a lab technician. Again, a test is inconclusive. The blood gas levels indicate that the baby is making some respiratory effort. Ryan does not have a hypoplastic lung condition.

A few minutes after 7:00 P.M. Joe Ritiglia places a call to the mother of the baby. "I have to talk to you about your baby," he begins. "You saw him. I understand you expected this?" The woman replies in the affirmative. Ritiglia discusses the family history of bone problems with her and describes how Ryan's arms and legs seem fixed, paralyzed. "Hard to put it all together. We have some ideas. Do you remember if the baby was moving or kicking around?" She answers, not since five months. "Then the baby may not have moved his arms and legs for some time. There are things that go along with this absence of movement—thin ribs, abnormal lungs. Now there is some suggestion that the lungs are abnormal but not horrible." She asks whether the baby is breathing. "We have a tube down into his lungs and we are breathing for him now." Ritiglia tells her about Ryan's abnormally large head and the fact that the CAT scan suggests that the brain has not developed normally. "We don't know for sure. But there are a lot of things that tell us that your baby has something wrong with his legs. Arms and legs are repairable. But if the reason for these problems is that the brain is not normal, then . . ." Mrs. Flynn asks how they will know for sure. "Time will show us that," Ritiglia answers. She asks what should be done. "It's not an easy decision to make right now." The woman adds that a cousin was born with brain damage. "That fits," Ritiglia responds. "Having that in your family helps fill out the picture. The question is, what to do. I can't make that decision because I don't know what the right or wrong thing is to do." Mrs. Flynn confesses to uncertainty also. "All right. Think on it."

At this point in the conversation Mr. Flynn gets on the phone. "We're not 100 percent sure what's going on," Ritiglia tells him. Then he redescribes the baby's condition to Mr. Flynn. "The ribs and bones are very thin on the X-ray. There are a number of diseases that cause paralysis at birth. That's right. Yes. Well, the brain either was not built right, or there was an injury and the brain shrank. No.

I can't say for sure from this that he will be retarded." The father asks if Ritiglia can tell him the cause of his son's paralysis. "That's a very difficult question. My gut reaction is that either the brain was not built right or it was an injury—and that caused the paralysis. We can get a consult. But I think he would be in the same situation we are in. Now let me drop the final thing on you. The lungs are not developed. And I don't know if he can live with his lungs. The question is, where do we go from here? What do we do? I know this is a lot to drop on you. I can understand how your wife . . ." Mr. Flynn asks what they can do for the baby. "We're a special care unit. We take crummy lungs and make them good. Or we try to. The question is, should we? If we ventilate him, then we can see whether his lungs will hold out." Mr. Flynn asks about treating the bone problems. "The arms and legs can be repaired. But if the problem is caused by the brain . . . Okay, okay. What we'll do is try to get a neurologist in the morning and see what he says." Mr. Flynn asks about the extent of treatment. "It will be an all-or-nothing thing," Ritiglia answers. "If he makes it tonight—his lungs are the thing. We'll know more if his lungs hold out tonight . . . Okay. So give us a call in the morning. And I'll call you tonight if anything happens . . . Okay. Just hang in there. Take care of yourself."

After Ritiglia hangs up the phone he begins musing about the parent's responses. "The father says, 'Do what you can.' So we'll put in an I.V. and go with it."

Later he and the other doctors profess disappointment with the Flynn's approach to their baby's problems. They talk about what an articulate educated parent would have done. Hunter says that such a parent would ask bluntly whether they are going to be burdened with ten years of a machine-dependent child. Ritiglia believes that "parents want a mental-retardation scale with their child located on it. They don't want probabilities." I think to myself that probabilities require decisions in conditions of uncertainty. Those are hard decisions. Bill Wade leans back in his chair. "I disagree. Parents are comfortable with probabilities. They hear such projections all the time—on TV weather shows, war games, games shows of all sorts." Ritiglia is doubtful. "They still want a retardation scale. And it doesn't exist." All of the doctors agree that smart parents would be inquisitive about their own burdens in the years ahead.

Rating parents is a common practice among doctors. As common as the practice are the egoistic principles used in the ratings. A parent who guards himself against being stuck with a totally dependent child who cannot respond to stimuli is admired by the doctors.

Such a parent displays a nice blend of prescience and pragmatism that impresses doctors. They are not impressed by parents who buy into situations without thinking of their long-term self-interest. Such parents are not altruists to the doctors but thoughtless people who do not appreciate the enormous burdens of caring for unresponsive infants.

2

May 10. Ryan is doing poorly. He is on a ventilator and the settings have to stay up to 34 at 100 percent oxygen just to keep him going. Even at those settings his blood gases are poor. Randy Hunter is pessimistic. "We're running out of guns to use. We've also given him prostaglandins to open him up. But he's still slipping." The doctors have discovered that Ryan has PFC as well (persistant fetal circulation). Real problems here.

An anomalous touch: "Magic. You can do magic" is playing on one of the radios in the nursery at this moment. "You can have anything that you desire. Magic."

Ryan's skin is unusually pink. He is seizing—while on phenobarbital. The tag over his bed reads "Baby boy Flynn" (no first name). Surrounding Ryan's crib are many of the routine yet magical machines of the nursery: a pneumogram (to keep track of respiratory rates), blood pressure recorders, a machine to monitor heart rates, a warmer, a transcutaneous monitor (to measure oxygen levels in the blood), machines to set rates of intraveneous fluids flowing into Ryan's bloodstream, and a ventilator.

Joe Ritiglia calls the Flynns again (it is noon). "Mrs. Flynn. this is Dr. Ritiglia. I thought I would fill you in on the night—what's been going on. Ryan is at 100 percent oxygen. Something else is going on in his lungs." Mrs. Flynn asks Ritiglia to talk to her husband. "Okay . . . I was explaining that he has come through the night, but not very easily. We've had the ventilator settings up. Also we've had some problems with something that goes along with small lungs— blood supply to lungs. We've had to go to hyperventilation— breathing real fast. There was an initial response, but Ryan is slipping back now to what he was. The next step was a medication, which has some bad effects. So we did that. Now we're doing all we can. So far he's hanging in there. Not great, but—but we've just about reached the end of our bag of tricks. What we'll see now is him slowly getting worse. A neurologist will be over this afternoon." Mr. Flynn asks if the neurologist will be able to help matters.

"No—he might be able to say what caused the whole thing—whether in the brain primarily or something else. But if the lungs don't get better there's nothing we can do . . . Right." Mr. Flynn asked about the point to the tests being run. "You might like to know if it's inherited," Ritigla tells him. Mr. Flynn volunteers some information. His mother had twins once that died. "Is that right? From what? . . . Were they premature?" Mr. Flynn answers that they were perfectly natural babies. "No," Ritigla points out, "natural babies live. So something was going on. . . . Well, if we figure out what it is, then you might know your chances for future babies . . . Well, I don't think anything is going to happen in a second. I'll call you this afternoon—maybe we'll know better then." Mr. Flynn asks what would be the normal levels of oxygen in a baby's blood. "The normal oxygen in the blood is 500. It was 20 to 40 this morning. The changes you see—with 100 percent oxygen you go to 500. He went from 20 to 40. So it's not good." Mr. Flynn asks what a life-support system is. "What they mean by life-support systems is you're breathing for him, giving fluids, and so on." Has Ryan been fed orally? "No, we haven't given anything to him orally." Mr. Flynn relates a story about a nurse telling them that Ryan was now eating. "And she said he was getting water, and something to eat?" Ritiglia questions. "No, we haven't given him anything by mouth. He has a tube in his stomach to empty air out. And we may have put fluid down the tube to clean it out. He gets all his nourishment through a vein." Mr. Flynn asks how sick Ryan is. "He's as sick as you can possibly be and still live. If he gets any sicker, he will not live . . . It's hard to know this unless you're in the field. And hard to tell a friend—you tend to make it a little better . . . I'll let you know. Things are getting worse. Okay. Goodbye." The conversation has lasted fifteen minutes.

Over in Stephanie's room time seems to be standing still. She is the same. The routines of treatment are the same. The staff seems to be reenacting a small drama whose point escapes all who witness it. At the moment Stephanie seems cooler and less restless than she normally is. She may at last be slowing down. Or she may simply be filled with morphine.

An intern raises an interesting question about Ryan Flynn. "I don't know why they called in a neurologist. The CAT scan showed enough brain to live. Whether there is enough for anything else no one knows. But to me its clear-cut—treat. The big issue now is whether he has enough lung tissue to live."

Joe Ritiglia comes over to respond. "We called in a neurologist to confirm diagnosis. It won't make any difference on treatment right now. But the parents would like to know what's wrong."

"Then he's coming in more for diagnosis than prognosis," the intern observes.

"Right."

I ask Ritiglia if Ryan's father understands what is happening.

"I don't know. It's hard to say. The less I think he understands, the blunter I get in describing the situation."

It is mid-afternoon. Ryan has a pneumothorax. The doctors succeed in getting a tube in his chest to keep the lungs inflated. Ryan is very pale. The PFC clamps down the vessels and interrupts blood to the lungs. Ryan's oxygen level is down to 9. Bill Camisa had said earlier today that Ryan would soon declare himself one way or the other. Apparently he has—negatively.

Camisa is looking at the X-ray photos. "This pneumo-thorax is very unusual. Very small." Apparently Ryan is consistently anomalous.

The new blood gas tests come back from the lab. Ryan now has an oxygen level of 7.4 with maximum ventilator support (100 percent oxygen at the highest possible settings). This is an oxygen level incompatible with life. (Even premies have an oxygen level of 50.) Camisa suctions Ryan's trachea, checks his mouth to make sure there are no obstructions. Then he inspects the intubation tube. Satisfied that there is no more to be done, he stands near Ryan's crib with his arms folded, staring down at the baby. Ryan is turning slowly darker. His feet are blue. He is absolutely inert.

A resident physician, a woman, asks, "Philosophically—was the baby baptized?"

A nurse nearby thinks he was.

The resident explains that if you do it and say nothing, no big deal. But if the mother freaks out afterwards on the realization that the baby was not baptized, then you can say, oh yes he was.

Someone tells Camisa that the neurologist in to see Ryan this morning thinks the child's condition may be a variant on trisomy 18. All of the neonatologists were skeptical. But Camisa, after a moment of thought, rushes off to order chromosomal tests.

I ask him when he returns if he would turn off Ryan's ventilator.

"Not in today's climate," he answers. "But if the parents were here we might try to speed things up when the heart rate starts dropping." Ryan's heart rate is 140 per minute right now. Camisa explains that the baby is probably in no discomfort. But if the parents were here, they would be suffering. The staff, he points out, tries to be merciful.

"We're just waiting it out right now," Camisa tells a nurse who has just come on her shift.

The nurse asks if he wants to run a test on Ryan's blood gases.

"No," he tells her. "No point. We can't do anything if they're bad." He turns to me and says that there will be no feeling of loss around here with this one. "Most people will be glad when it's over."

The doctors and nurses drift away from Ryan's bed to tend to other babies. Ryan keeps turning progressively darker. His eyes are slits.

I drift away also, my movements turning (as always) in the direction of the opposite wing of the nursery and Stephanie's room. She is being suctioned by a nurse. Blood is coming up. Stephanie's face is swollen, bruised. She looks old. Every time the tube is inserted in her mouth and nasal passages she cries. The nurse is being very gentle. But it is still agony.

Kevin Scott, an intern, comes over to look in on Stephanie. He tells me that one problem in medical care today is that our society has no plan for the dying. What can you do, he asks rhetorically, when a child is terminal? "Here, Mrs. Jones. Take home your child. Feed every three hours, use Ivory soap, and watch him die in two weeks." You can't say that, Scott tells me. But there is no other way that makes any sense either. Scott believes that people are isolated today from the old and the dying. The result is an impoverishment of human experience. Scott also stresses, as others on the staff have again and again, the things that doctors can do in therapy to kill a baby. Already, he notes, Ryan is in the danger zone from treatment alone. Risk and benefit must be in balance. The respirator, Scott feels, cannot be increased much beyond 34 in these circumstances without destroying Ryan's lungs.

We walk over together back to Ryan's crib. "That kid in there is turning black," a resident observes as she leaves the room where Ryan is being treated. A nurse suggests that a cardiologist be called in to see Ryan. This proposal meets with no enthusiasm.

Ritiglia is standing near Ryan's bed. "We're letting nature take its course."

I ask Ritiglia if anyone has considered turning off the ventilator. "No," he answers. "Letting things go is one thing. Acting in a negative way is another. But if the parents were here and wanted to stop treatment—definitely. I would stop treatment."

Someone asks where Ryan's father is.

"He's out on business," Ritiglia answers.

"He's also out of touch," a nurse responds. Another asks what business could be more important than a dying child. The Flynns, I learn, have no other children. They are in their mid-twenties.

A nurse comes over and covers Ryan with a white diaper. She explains that another baby in the room will be coming back from surgery soon accompanied by his mother. "And the mother is kind of fainty." Ryan is breathing rapidly. Only the top of his head is not covered. His eyes are still half-open.

At 4:45 P.M. Ryan's heart rate starts to jump around, from 133 to 130 to 129. Fifteen minutes later his heart rate is down to 88.

Ritiglia calls Mrs. Flynn and, in a short but compassionate conversation, tells her that "it's just a matter of time now. Probably within hours." The mother tells Ritiglia that her husband cannot be there at the hospital. She asks that a photograph be taken of her baby.

Everyone starts looking for a camera. A nurse slides the diaper covering off Ryan. There is a small deposit of stool at his anus. The nurse considers this and decides aloud not to wipe him off. Then she changes her mind. She gently cleans Ryan and changes the diaper on which he is resting.

At ten minutes after 5:00 P.M., Ryan's heart rate is 54. It is falling rapidly—down to 37 one minute later. A nurse listens to Ryan's heart with a stethoscope. The heart rate is now 27.

Someone comes into the room and announces that transport has a camera. It is located in a little room downstairs. A nurse leaves the nursery to get it. Ryan's heart rate is 11.

"Looks like it's about over," Jay O'Brien observes. He has just seen Ryan for the first time.

The nurse returns with the camera. "Should I take it with all the tubes in?"

O'Brien reflects on this question. "Well. Most of them have to stay in."

The nurse can't figure out how to work the polaroid camera. Kevin Scott takes the camera from her and photographs Ryan with all of the tubes in place. A nurse accidentally spills a jar of sterile water on the floor across the room. The staff around Ryan's bed glance over at the accident and then resume watching Ryan. There is much favorable comment about the quality of the developing photograph. Scott takes a second, much closer to the baby, of Ryan's head.

At 5:30 P.M. the baby who has been at surgery returns with a retinue of doctors and nurses. The parents trail behind the group.

Ryan's heart rate drops to 4 per minute, then jumps up to 34, then down to 20. A young physician from the surgery group comes over to Ryan's crib and lifts up the diaper for a look. He calls the chief surgeon, Dr. West, over to look. West tells him in hushed tones, "He has an O_2 level of 7." The young physician is astounded. "Seven?" he echoes. West nods. They both move away, back to the crib of their patient.

The nurse attending to Ryan removes the baby's ventilator tube momentarily. Ryan's heart rate sinks to 1, with no respiration. She reinserts the tube. At 5:40 P.M. the nurse cannot hear anything through the stethoscope. She calls O'Brien over. He listens. At 5:42 P.M. O'Brien removes the stethoscope and says there is nothing. No heartbeat. He removes the ventilator tube and asks if chromosomes were drawn for tests. Yes, they were. That's it. Baby Flynn is dead.

Ritiglia calls Mrs. Flynn and tells her that Ryan has expired. "And that was that," he says. O'Brien fills out the death certificate. The cause of death is a common one: cardiac-pulmonary arrest, in turn caused by pulmonary hypoplasia caused by multiple congenital anomalies. Born 13:13 on May 9. Died 18:42 on May 10.

Ryan's body is being cleaned up in the privacy of the treatment room. He was removed quickly from room A because of the presence of the parents of the surgical baby. Later Ryan will be taken downstairs to the morgue by the nurses. A nurse is trying to take another photo of Ryan, this time with all tubes and wires removed and the baby propped up on its side with a diaper wrapped up to his chin. The bulb flashes. I close the door and leave, with a picture of inert Ryan in my head as a last memory—clean, unsmiling, though attractive in a way that one hopes will serve his parents' needs.

An average of two babies a week die in Northeastern's special care nursery. Each death is different. But, in general, death is not an awesome event in young babies with severe problems. Ryan, to the staff, never really began his life. The emotions of death seem to occur among sentient and thoughtful human beings. The absence of Ryan's parents removed most of those emotions from the scene of his demise. He did not live long enough to enter the contract of human relations found in the nursery.

Outside the hospital I see people walking in bright sun with a cooling breeze. Is there any doubt that forms of living, of human life, are, finally, cultivated arts? Simply being in existence is not a human life. Contributing in some way to human practices, even when as passive as Stephanie's life, is what we mean by human existence.

3

May 11. Early in the morning. I am working at home when a call comes from the hospital. A nurse taking care of Stephanie tells me that she died at 4:02 A.M. this morning. The cause of death was recorded as cardiac arrest. The parents have donated her eyes to the organ bank. The fight is over.

I go into my younger daughter's bedroom. Everywhere there are signs of achievement, of art and sensibility. Chrissy holding a math trophy in a photograph. Sketches, poems, short stories on the dresser and floor. Stephanie Christopher lived nine weeks and part of a day in a special care nursery. She didn't even know the effects she had on everyone who came into contact with her. Or how much some people became attached to her.

> *From an interview with the nurse who was caring for Stephanie at her death.*

Frohock: Can you tell me about Stephanie's death?

Nurse: Let's see. She was pink all night long. She'd been pink all evening long. At 3:00 I went in, suctioned her out, turned her over. She was pink. At 3:15 I looked in the window. She was pink. Twenty, twenty-five after three, she wasn't pink anymore. She was gray. She wasn't breathing.

We went into the room. She had a heart rate of 45, 50. She was gray. Totally unresponsive. Suctioned her out thinking her airway was occluded. There was nothing in her airway. Stimulated her physically, you know, hitting her feet, gently shaking her bed. There was no response. We called the doc. At this point, she'd already been in 100 percent oxygen blowing in her face. We just made sure it was right up in her face some more. The charge nurse was on. She called the doctor. He came down and we gave her narcan. We gave her one dose of narcan and there was no response, so we just let her go. At that point, her heart rate was 35 and she was totally unresponsive. She was still unresponsive after the narcan. So it was probably between 3:30, quarter of four and at 4:00 we didn't hear a heart rate anymore. Her color—she never got responsive. She never gasped. She never did anything. Her heart rate just kept slowing and she never breathed. She'd gotten morphine at 2:00, but this was 3:30 and usually morphine peaks in a hour or so and the narcan would have reversed it. It didn't. So she just went.

Frohock: Now that we've seen what happened, did it make sense to treat this baby at all?

Nurse: I think you had to treat her. I think it was wise that we weren't any more aggressive than we'd been towards the end, because although her skin healed, she also got new blisters every few days. It was a never-ending cycle of healing and breaking down and the possibility of infection was always, always there. It never got better. It was just kind of a cycle that didn't get broken. So I think you had to treat her, but I think we were right in not being aggressive. I mean, when you look at statistics, this type of disease is not one that you generally live with.

Frohock: What was the hardest thing for you in treating her?

Nurse: Just the frustration, that she was in pain. The last couple days I'd had her, even with morphine, you went to touch her and she'd whimper. She just never seemed comfortable, and we had to change her dressings. You couldn't ignore her and you knew that every time you did them she was going to hurt. She was going to cry and she was going to kick. Half the time she might kick the dressings off so you'd have to repeat the whole process again. It was just frustration more than anything else.

Frohock: What was your feeling when she died?

Nurse: I don't know. I wasn't upset. It was just kind of—it had been coming. She'd been trying off and on for a few weeks to stop breathing. Her heart rate would drop and then we'd get her stimulated and she'd come back. It just was kind of like—it just surprised me that it happened so fast. Within five minutes, she'd gone from glowing and pink to gray with no heart rate. I think that was the worst, just the shock that it happened so fast.

From an interview with Kevin Scott, the intern on duty when Stephanie died.

Scott: What time was this? About 3:00 in the morning they called me to see her. She wasn't breathing very well and she was just gasping intermittently, not making regular respirations, and her heart rate was down. She was given morphine for pain about an hour before that and one thing morphine can do is slow the heart down and slow respirations down. So I gave her an antidote to the morphine, narcan, because that was the plan beforehand. It was already made. The decision was made. So I gave her that and I didn't do anything. Then I pretty much walked away, because there was nothing else to do. She had the O_2. She had the oxygen flowing to her face. She wasn't bleeding from anywhere. The plan was not to give her any medication to speed her heart rate up and we were not going to do any chest compressions on her or intubate her, so there was nothing else to do.

When we gave the narcan, I knew if she lived that in the morning I would get yelled at half in jest for giving it to her—half in earnest. The nurses didn't want to give it to her that night and I definitely didn't rush to give it to her. For one thing, I didn't think it made a difference because it was a very symbolic thing giving it to her or not giving it to her at that point. She had gotten the morphine so far beforehand that I didn't think it could be that at all. I gave her the narcan anyway, I guess because it was ordained that that was not going to be the way she was going to die, from a morphine overdose. There are many people who die from an intentional morphine overdose. They're in such intense pain, you just give them morphine and morphine until they have no more pain. But for some reason, she wasn't going to die that way. I don't think that's what she died from anyway because the time course wasn't right. When she died we—it's always wonderful having somebody die on you, if he's not your patient, in the middle of the night. I knew what was going on with her, but it would have been better if a resident had been there. I called surgery and they called Dr. West. He called the parents and I went back to bed.

Then the mom called up. This was probably about 4–4:30 and they got me out of bed. The nurse says, "The mom wants to donate the eyes," and I'm half asleep. So I speak to the mom and I said—I'd seen her a lot but I never really talked to her before—and I said, "the nurses tell me that you want to donate the eyes." And she said, "No. I was just talking with my dad and we want you people to study her body so you can learn about the disease." And I said "Well, would you like to donate the eyes, because no matter what size the baby is, they could use the cornea." She said "Yes." And then I said, "Do you want an autopsy? Is that what you're saying?" She said, "I don't know, speak to my dad." The grandfather got on the phone and he said, "I want you people to take the body and study the body and learn something about this disease. You don't know a damn thing about it." He didn't say it in a bad way, he said it in a truthful way; and I said, "Well, that's an autopsy." He said, "Sure. Whatever you want. Keep the body two or three weeks and study it." And I almost started laughing. I said "Well, we only need it for like a day or so." He said "No, no. You keep it, three weeks, a month, whatever. We don't need it. Just give it back when you're done." I did all I could to not laugh. That was basically the end of it and then signing the death certificate.

From an interview with a second nurse who had treated Stephanie.
Nurse: She had to have a lot of dressing changes. She sort of reminded me a little bit of a burn patient. People who take care of burn patients or patients that are in a lot of pain say that at the time of treatment of course the patients are going to say that they want to die because their treatments are very painful. In a baby, you don't even have the option of knowing what they think or what they say because they can't tell you. At least not in words. She was on a lot of morphine because she was in a lot of pain. From that respect alone, I don't know if what we were doing was always so great. Her dressing changes and stuff seemed to be pretty painful as best we could tell—again, because she was only a baby. I, at least, believed that she was in pain for part of the time anyway. Her skin was quite often just open sores. She bled a lot. She had a lot of problems with keeping her platelet count up for various reasons, and because of that, she had a lot of oozing, a lot of bleeding, a lot of open scabs and stuff where the blisters were. She was alert and awake most of the time, at times agitated, again we presume because she was in pain. But she acted like a pretty normal baby, I thought, for the most part.

I guess that was sort of hard for most people. Because she acted so normal, I think that she could let us know that she was in pain and that things hurt. That was sort of upsetting, I think, to the people who had to take care of her. I saw her maybe once or twice a day. I usually would go in there every day, but I wasn't one of the nurses who had to work with her for eight hours and change her dressings, etc. I really have a lot more admiration for them since they had to be the ones to be in there. There was one incident. I was called down to see her early one morning and she had stopped breathing. She'd had an apneic episode and just wouldn't breathe for about three or four minutes, just wouldn't take a breath. On the front of her chart was her code status, worked out by her attending physician with the mother and father, listing the things that we weren't supposed to do—we were not supposed to intubate her, give her any vasoactive meds like epinephrine, or give her cardiac compressions. At the time I went down there for the apneic episode, we ended up giving her a little positive pressure. Just two or three breaths to see if she would come around. And we finally ended up giving her some narcan. Since she was on morphine, we thought maybe things had built up. We gave her that and she seemed to come around. I found out the next day that the nurses on night shift were very upset that we had given her the narcan. I guess as much as I felt like she should be allowed to die or whatever, that I was not going to allow it to be because of an overdose of morphine. I didn't really think that that was right somehow. If we're going to do that, then let's just say we're doing that and give her as much morphine as she wants. But since we're saying that we're going to take care of her and do what we can for her, then I didn't think that was appropriate.

On the night that she died I know they did give her narcan again and it seemed to have no effect. It sounds like she died of a similar episode—kind of stopped breathing and dropped the heart rate, etc. It's interesting. I saw the mother the day after. We had to go down to sign an autopsy permit. She's going to have a tubal. She's not going to have any more children. I think it was sad all around. In terms of whether it was worth it, I don't know if anybody could really say what's worth it. I don't know. She spent her whole life in the hospital. She spent a large part of it, I think, in pain. But if she had been that rare kid who made it, then I guess it would have been worth it. So you're always obligated to try. She got treated several times on antibiotics. We did certain minimal things for her.

I guess I don't feel bad about any of the things that we did for her in prolonging her agony. But on the other hand I wasn't overly upset when I found out that she had died. I was upset that the situation had occurred, but I felt like in a way that she was being relieved of some of this agony that she was going through. I think it was also very stressful on the nurses who had to take care of her. Not only was it physically stressful—the room was very hot because of her temperature instability and that sort of thing. They talked a lot about that. But I think part of it was the stress of just having to take care of her in and of itself, just sort of a displacement of their feelings.

From an interview with Bill Wade

Frohock: If you could go back in time, run the film back, and you had complete control of Stephanie's treatment, what would you have done at the beginning?

Wade: I would not have brought in any extra resources. I think that's the major difference where I would have departed from what did happen. I certainly would have provided nutrition, would have treated with antibiotics, would have done much of the skin debriding. But I probably wouldn't have flown in the bed. I would have taken the child to the bed. We're not capable of using that bed.

Frohock: Did the bed make a difference?

Wade: I don't think so.

Frohock: It may have prolonged her life?

Wade: Prolonged it. It's one of those unfortunate diseases where there still is no defined therapy. Most anything that's been done thus far has been buying time. Sooner or later someone will come up with a medication or combination of medications that's effective. But this particular medical center, with that sort of metabolic disease, is not going to be the place to do it. We just don't have the horses.

From an interview with Roger West, the primary physician in the treatment of Stephanie.

Frohock: Was the effort worth it, all things considered?

West: The effort was probably not worth it. But I think the problem that comes up is that any time somebody says that one of these patients with this particular skin disease had survived, it puts you in a bind. You almost cannot refuse what you feel is a reasonable amount of medical care. You're in a situation where if there's any hope at all, you have to at least try. And I think that's what is going to cause the difficulties in the years to come. People will start rationing medical care on the basis of cost and they are going to basically use percentages. That's the only way to make those kind of decisions and it's going to be a disaster. There's no question it's going to be a disaster.

Frohock: What roughly are the percentages?

West: I think in that particular case the dermatologist told me of only one or two patients that he knew that had survived. Now, I think in that particular instance we tried for several weeks. When it became obvious that we were not going to succeed, we backed off with some of the care. But I don't think at that particular point—I can't stop feeding the baby. I just can't do that. So you give some basic medical care. But if the baby has a cardiac arrest you don't resuscitate her. If they get pneumonia, you probably would not go all out to treat them. Those kinds of things. I think that's more of a passive-type thing than an active type of thing. I think with that particular infant we probably tried for a good several weeks and it rapidly became obvious that we were not going to be successful.

Frohock: When you determined that you were not going to be successful, did that mean in your mind that that baby would not survive?

West: Yes, yes, yes, and my feeling was that it was 100 percent. I think that's going to be part of the problem. In other words, if you're not at 100 percent, what numbers do you use? Do you stop at 85 percent, 90 percent, 95 percent, and who determines that? You know as a physician that you've taken an oath that you're going to do everything you can. You don't take an oath that says you're going to do everything you can if it's 85 percent valid. Now, if it's 100 percent that you're not going to succeed, than you have an obligation to make that patient as comfortable as you can and do the best for the family you can. But there is that gray zone in between that is very difficult. I find it exceedingly difficult.

I asked West in the course of the interview how much Stephanie's suffering affected the staff after they had decided that the baby could not survive.

West: We did give that baby a lot of morphine. It bothered us very much. Again, there's no question that you can take a baby like that and give them an overdose of potassium. There are any one of a number of ways to do something about that. If the family would agree, I would think that would be a reasonable thing to do. Unfortunately, with the laws in the United States we can't do that. In a nursery situation we cannot take a chance and do that. We just cannot do that. You're risking a lot. If somebody doesn't agree with what you do, you will have the district attorney breathing down your neck very rapidly. So while we certainly do use some forms of passive euthanasia in such situations, we really don't use active euthanasia. I don't do anything actively to speed the demise of infants. But the pain and suffering bothers anyone involved in those situations. And for that reason we used an awful lot of morphine for such a little baby.

Frohock: Suppose the parents had wanted to bring the experience to a close on humanitarian impulses. Is there anything—is there any gray zone between active and passive euthanasia that hospital staff could employ?

West: Yes. In certain instances. Not with this baby. But we have had babies on ventilators per se that if all parties are agreeable, not only the parents and the physicians but including the nursing staff, if all parties agree, we have taken patients off ventilators. Now that's something that actually in New York State is really against the law because these patients have not been what we call brain dead. They are not brain dead. We do that because I have felt that in those situations the baby will succumb within twelve hours, say, if we leave the baby on the ventilator. And I just cannot see prolonging the misery of the entire situation. We have done that. Unfortunately, the particular baby that you're talking about did not lend itself to that method. I can't see myself coming in with a syringe full of something and injecting it into the baby's veins, for instance. I can't see myself at this point. At some point in the future, I actually think that's what's going to happen and I would do it. I honestly would do it, because there are certain places for that.

From an interview with Kevin Scott

Frohock: Now, in retrospect, did it make sense to treat her at all?

Scott: To have treated her at all? Well, sure. We didn't know at the beginning what was going to happen to her. We knew it'd be difficult and the odds were very slim, but she might have made it. I don't know. Most likely not. Economically it didn't make sense, but I guess it doesn't make sense to treat most people economically. I think that some administrators would be happy if we just closed everything down and kept an empty building because that way we wouldn't lose that much money. She was probably in pain a good amount of time. I don't know how much in terms of what she got out of her life. She didn't do much different than the other premies, which is pretty much just kind of lie there and look around once in a while. Whether that's significant in the scheme of things, probably not. The same way an amoeba floating around isn't all that important one way or the other. But it was her life, I guess. It was all she had. Her family, I would think, benefited from her. And I'm sure there are a lot of scars from it. The people here are the same way. I think there are a lot of scars from her being here, but I think they also benefited from her. A lot of how we benefit from these kids is just being thankful that there are healthy ones. I don't know if it's worth it to put somebody through torture for three months just to realize that, but that's definitely a benefit from a lot of what I see around here. It's so sad. And it makes you very fearful of anybody you know having a baby and very thankful when they come out okay. Like I said, I don't know if it's worth somebody going through torture for three months to get that through your head. I don't know, if you balanced it all out, exactly which way the scales would tip. But I think there's enough on the positive side and enough doubt that you've got to keep doing it anyway. I guess that's the bottom line.

4

A vision of the individual dominates (some would say haunts) western traditions. It is sketched out on the thought that human beings are isolated rational units, separate from each other and from the larger society that they somehow constitute. The thought begins in modern terms with the contract theorists of the seventeenth and eighteenth centuries. It continues through utilitarianism in the nineteenth and twentieth centuries. Today the thought informs wide stretches of economic and social theory. Recent democratic practices are nourished on the proposition that the single individual, the individual simpliciter, is the rock-bottom foundation of society—origin and judge of all value in the world. Society itself is often said to be derived from, and reducible to, individuals. Nothing exists but individuals.

No one working in special care nurseries can hold on to that vision. To embrace it is to court insanity. For if individuals are the focus for reality and value, then the infants who live and die like Ryan Quinn and Stephanie Christopher have no meaning or place in the world. The Quinn baby lived just over thirty hours. Stephanie lived a life of continual pain whose duration was slightly more than nine weeks. If we use a test drawn from thoroughgoing individualism to evaluate life—its quality to an individual—these two lives make no sense at all. They had no quality in these terms. So long as individuals are the primary sources for meaning and value, the treatment of a Stephanie Christopher is unintelligible.

A longer tradition of social thought provides a different vision. Classical philosophers celebrate the community over the individual. Both Plato and Aristotle view the group as the primary unit of human existence. Individuals exist as members of larger contexts, not separate from those communities that are the conditions for human life. The meaning of Stephanie Christopher's life, seen within this view, is not found in its quality for Stephanie. It is rather to be found in the human communities in terms of which Stephanie has human status. These are hard moves to make. It is not easy to say that Stephanie's pain is justified by the effects she had on others. Certainly there is no sense to this judgment (as Kevin Scott saw) if Stephanie's life merely heightens our gratitude at having normal children. Yet unless some broader reference is introduced, some sense of Stephanie's location in a larger scheme of things, neither Stephanie's life nor her treatment make any sense.

Special care communities seems to be driven by conflicting rules and principles. Many of the imperatives to treat are drawn from the individualistic languages of recent social theory. Individuals are said to have rights to medical care, treatment is to be organized for the best interests of the individual patient, the quality of life to an individual is important, and so on. Many of these principles of care are left to the individual to interpret. This is a logic impeccable in its consistency with individualistic traditions, since these traditions accept the individual as the origin of value (especially as these values bear on his own life). But the patients in neonatal units are not the individuals assumed in recent social thought. They are not rational, not competent to make those decisions that individuals must make if medical care is to remain within individualistic traditions. So the driving rules and principles of medicine falter, break down. The staffs are left with a language (of rights, interests, quality) that cannot be used in the way it is typically used—as an instrument to disclose what is of value to autonomous individuals.

The two cases—Ryan Quinn and Stephanie Christopher—illustrate the ways in which special care staffs accommodate the deficiencies of individualistic languages. Viability is the beginning supplement. Babies often "declare themselves," meaning that they make a kind of decision to live or die early on. Ryan Quinn presented no special problems for the staff, for he was a nonviable child. Many babies do expire no matter how they are treated. But viability tests do not solve all of the problems in the nursery. Stephanie Christopher fought for her life even though the outcome of her battle was virtually preordained. In these cases, the staff puts together a mosaic of decisions involving families (parents, especially) and staff to settle on the best course of treatment. Sometimes the decisions are rational and human by any standards. At other times they fail to meet any reasonable tests of reason and value (and fail in different ways—witness the Cutlass and Monihan babies). On still other occasions, as with Stephanie, there is no agreement on whether the right things were done even after the treatment has concluded.

A pragmatist would say that the language of medical practice needs adjustment. Some fine tuning of rights, interests, quality, can provide a conceptual endowment that will avoid ambivalence and failure. But perhaps the problems cut to a deeper level. It may be that our languages are inherently flawed when extended to medical care today, and that we need an entirely different framework to address issues in neonatology practices.

11
Languages of Evaluation

1

In the summer of 1984 an American couple flew to Australia for a type of in vitro fertilization. The woman's ova were artificially fertilized by her husband's sperm outside her womb, and then the fertilized ova were allowed to grow in a laboratory. Unfortunately the couple was killed in a plane crash before the fertilized ova could be implanted in the woman's uterus. Authorities were faced with the question of what to do with the frozen embryos that remained (in a kind of suspended state). At first the problem was framed as an issue in property law. The couple had left no instructions on how to dispose of something that they owned. Then resistance grew to any thought of destroying the embryos. They began to be seen as the living progeny of the couple. Some began discussing the right to life of the embryos and the need to implant them in some other woman's uterus in order to allow them to gestate and be born.

Many ironies heighten the strangeness of these events. One is that Locke's coupling of property rights (over one's body) and the right of self-preservation is renewed, though in unusual ways. Can we own our progeny *and* invest them simultaneously with a right to life? Another is the tortured stretching of inheritance law that will occur if these embryos are implanted and born. A tradition of law that marks off progeny from one another may have to admit to the commonality of human experience in recognizing a child born to a surrogate mother as the heir to a family unrelated to the woman by blood or marriage. But the one impression from the events dominating all else is the anomalous connection of language to experience. To say that fertilized ova have rights to life is surely to stretch rights language to the breaking point.

The language of rights originates in modern form in the contract theories of the seventeenth and eighteenth centuries. Hobbes and

Locke broke with long traditions of medieval law that located sovereignty in law. They chose instead to assign sovereignty to individuals. Individuals were to have rights to preserve themselves and to defend their own lives (Hobbes and Locke) and to freedom and property (Locke). Such rights seal off individuals from social regulation, establishing zones of autonomy within which individuals are sovereign in their actions. The philosophy, however, demands certain powers of individuals. Individuals must be rational. They must be responsible for their actions. They must in general be able to exercise the authority over their own lives that was formerly located in social practices.

Such expectations for individuals suggest an ambitious level of knowledge. Rights language was originally formed on the premise that we know what a human being is. Humans were said to be rational and autonomous creatures who, on the basis of such powers, are assigned rights of various sorts. Historically, rights are possessed by adult males (white adult males who own property, to make the point more finely). Children, for example, were not granted rights of any importance until recently. The one exception is a right to life (itself a recent historical construction). But even this right is developed on the premise that its possessor has certain sentient qualities, chief among these the capability now or in the future for making conscious choices in a rational and free manner. We do not assign rights to life even to higher vertebrates because we believe that such creatures lack the capacities for sovereign action that humans possess more or less routinely.

The staff at the nursery use rights language. They admit that all of the babies have a right to life, "the same right as you or I have." But they are also troubled that this right is assigned to infants who, in their judgment, ought not to be kept alive. Part of the trouble they sense here may be due to the effects of rights language in medical communities. In the nursery a right to life is used as a compensation for the failure of individual sovereignty. Those infants who do not have, and will never have, those very capacities that traditionally mark off the human species as a bearer of a right to life are sometimes kept alive by the medical community as a kind of good-faith endorsement of life itself. The original idea of a right is changed by such efforts. A right in traditional social thought, unlike a law, is a shield insulating the individual from regulation by others without (as a law does) obligating the individual to any action. A right to life thus means that no one may take the life of one who has that right (at least without justification). The right does not require its bearer to stay alive. When institutions keep people alive without any test to determine whether they would accept the conditions of their lives, the right to life has been transformed into an obligation to live—which is not a right at all.

The deeper puzzlement expressed by the staff, however, seems to be produced by a conflict between their humanitarian impulses and the actions required by right-to-life language. They feel strongly that the best thing to do in some circumstances is "pull a plug"—shut off a ventilator—or refuse to treat. The dignity of the patient is violated, they say, when he is kept alive "as a vegetable." It would be better to let him die. Yet they acknowledge that the patient's right to live blocks such efforts. The conflict they express is between the values they attach to individuals—dignity, autonomy, even the high standing of individual life found in liberal philosophies—and the rights that traditionally represent and protect those values.

The curious hold that rights language has on medical practice can be explained in many ways, most deriving from larger social needs and expectations imposed on medicine. Rights language is an effective instrument to bring about change in social practices. It is especially valuable whenever abuses must be corrected (and medical practice has not been free of such abuses—see the account of the syphilis experiments in James Jones's *Bad Blood*). More generally, rights protect individuals against community breakdowns. It is instructive to realize that a number of institutional forms, past and present, do not rely on rights to ensure the deeper values of dignity, autonomy, life. Small religious communities and intact families are among these types of institutions in modern societies. When these institutions break down, however, rights are powerful devices to ensure individual interests. Child abuse, for example, is probably more effectively addressed by assigning rights to children than by any other corrective method. But it is important to remember that rights are the instruments to represent deeper values, the conclusions of a hypothetical dialogue on the meaning and importance of individual life, not items valuable in themselves or simplistic trump cards to stop discourse on values. Seen in this way, a discussion of rights can admit the question—are there alternative instruments to realize the values we want rights to protect?

The staff at the nursery invoke a different language when they stress the importance of not harming patients with the advanced therapy they use. The Hippocratic oath's injunction to "do no harm" has a more general appeal than realized by the nursery staff.

Think for a moment of the Bloomington baby tragedy (arguably the worst of the recent medical neglect cases). Here parents refused to allow corrective surgery, and a child starved to death in a hospital. A right to life is not needed to avoid such horror. One would not starve a dog to death, yet dogs are not granted a right to life. A humanitarian impulse can avoid these events, expressible in an understanding that living creatures are not to be harmed in unreasonable ways.

The use of a harm principle may avoid the current extension of rights to types of life that are distant from the life forms on which rights languages were founded. Medical science today has created or disclosed forms of human life unknown to anyone living before the twentieth century. We now have frozen embryos and anencephalic babies, and are aware that life extends to them. Many (though not all) of these life forms do not meet the tests of conscious awareness traditionally used to justify assigning rights to life. Note that the life forms of this century may count as humans in a variety of communities. Humanness is not an issue. The issue is whether rights can be extended to life forms that do not in any important way resemble the individuals used to develop rights originally.

The error in extending rights language seems to be part of the failure to see the power of alternative languages to protect individuals. If frozen embryos do not have a right to life, then it may be thought there are no restriction on how they can be treated. But the concept of *harm* already carries into the discussion the suggestion of limits. The proposition that harm is to be avoided whenever possible can constrain actions, and because of its contextual qualities it can do so more credibly than a right-to-life shield. Not claiming the identity of all life forms when none can be established, a harm constraint can instead be concerned to disclose how particular forms of life are harmed and to draw constraints on action that are sensitive to differences among life forms.

2

Pain is a constant reminder in the nursery that all sentient forms of life can suffer. The babies are constantly subject to the routine pain of therapy—needles to draw blood, to start I.V. lines, to introduce antibiotics, even the nurse's daily thumpings of the babies to clear their trachea. There is also the pain of illness, illustrated in the extreme by Stephanie Christopher. Physical pain may dominate the range of pain in the nursery, though there is evidence that infants can also suffer emotional pains like fear, embarrassment, and humiliation. Older patients in hospitals may experience emotional pain that exceeds any physical pain they suffer.

Emotional pain can be a consequence of actions that offend either social convention or moral principles. A doctor who is curt with a patient offends propriety. He may cause a kind of mental discomfort that, while falling short of emotional pains like fear, is a painful experience. But offensive actions can also exceed conventions by violating rules drawn from moral principles. A hospital that requires a follower of the Jehovah's Witnesses to have a blood transfusion may save the patient's life by forcing him to violate his religious principles. There is no point arguing that the individual is better off alive, for many believe that certain principles are more important than life. Courts routinely affirm the importance of moral beliefs in establishing damages for mental anguish.

Both physical and emotional pain specify some of the ways in which individuals can be harmed. But there is another way individuals can be harmed. Suppose that the frozen embryos are destroyed. They would not suffer physical or emotional pain. They have no nervous system for pain. Nor do they have beliefs that can be offended. They can, however, suffer deprivation. To destroy them would be to deprive them of all possible future experiences. No one can doubt that this action would harm the embryos. They would have been denied the prospect of life itself.

The critical issue in using *harm* as a constraint on action is in determining how the three specifications—(a) physical pain, (b) emotional pain (through e.g., offensive actions), and (c) deprivation—actually count as harmful actions. Consider physical pain. To inflict pain on a baby through the use of an I.V. line is not to harm the baby. The physical pain is required in order to help the patient. If, on the other hand, an intern practices inserting I.V. needles on a patient time after time, this is pain for no therapeutic purpose. The patient is now harmed by the action. Or suppose that a patient is blocking an understanding of his physical condition through various defense mechanisms. A psychiatrist might judge that exposing the patient to emotional pain is the best vehicle to break through the defense in order to force the patient to confront his condition. If such confrontation is needed to begin effective therapy, then inflicting the emotional pain may be justifiable. The patient may be helped rather than harmed by the pain. Or suppose that a baby is born with trisomy 18. Not treating the baby may deprive him of some measurable time of life. But few would claim that the baby is harmed by such deprivation.

The consideration interpreting harm in these cases is the purpose of the action. What ends are the actions designed to achieve? An individual is harmed by physical pain, offensive actions, or deprivation only if such actions do not aim to restore some state of individual well-being. The determination of harm is not in medical communities a utilitarian calculation of benefits versus pain, offense, or deprivation. There *is* a consideration of benefits. And the benefits must exceed the suffering experienced for therapy to be worthwhile. But a classical concept of harm is more appropriate. Harm in the nursery is making something worse. Medical intervention is an effort to remove or reduce impediments to health. Therapy respects natural processes, and this respect requires physicians to forbear, to restrict actions. The opposite of harm is thus not, as in utilitarianism, doing or maximizing good, but rather allowing a teleological process to reach an end state.

The problem in using harm in this way is that the classical notion of function is not fixed in medical communities. A natural physiological state of well-being can be specified. Good health is a recognizable condition. But even this natural state of health is influenced by community values. The willingness of parents to accept and care for their infants, for example, affects the long-term health and even survival of the infant. Health is thus in part created by the attitudes of those intimately connected to a child. It is not a natural condition that develops according to laws independent of human influence. Also, no hierarchy of values is recognized by all members of the medical community. It is still possible (and indeed rational) for individuals to abandon health on the acceptance of alternative values. Suppose an individual stricken with a terminal disease for which there is no cure, only the chance to prolong life. It is not unreasonable (or atypical) for such an individual to forgo treatment in order to spare his family the agony of an extended death. In a case like this, deprivation is less harmful to the individual than therapy so long as he identifies his interests with those of his family.

The sensitivity of health to contextual considerations tells us again that therapy decisions are in some measure discretionary. Liberal thought assigns this discretionary power to the individual who is affected by decisions. Imagine deciding for a patient that he is to be denied life in order that his family can be spared the spectacle of his suffering. Liberal philosophers from Kant forward have demonstrated the moral error in using any human life as a means to secure the well-being of others. But even liberalism allows a competent individual, deciding for himself and with the ability to carry out his decisions, to introduce the interests of others in a determination of harm.

The problem in a neonatal nursery, of course, is that the patients are not competent by virtue of their age. But the task of determining individual harm when patients are incompetent is made easier by two considerations. The first is that some medical outcomes are clearly primary goods, meaning that they are valuable in themselves and desirable to virtually all rational individuals. Health is such a good. (Life may be a conditional good—desirable only on the satisfaction of other conditions, among which may be certain levels of health.) That patients want a restoration of health can be assumed without reconstructing the preferences of the individuals to be treated (though if the therapy is particularly painful or hazardous, some consideration of preferences may be needed). Health, on the whole, is an assumed goal in medical practice, capable of being overridden by other considerations but justified as a desirable end state in the absence of overriding considerations. Since infant children cannot provide such countervailing arguments, cannot consider subordinating health to other goals, the primary goal of medicine in restoring health is more firmly fixed in the nursery than in treating competent adults.

The second consideration is the form of life about which harm is to be determined. Life without a nervous system cannot be harmed by means of physical pain. Nor can life without the capacity for beliefs be harmed emotionally. On the same logic, a life incapable of conscious experiencing cannot suffer the same deprivation as a life without the possibility of consciousness. An anencephalic baby is not deprived of sentient life when treatment is withheld. An embryo in vitro is denied the future possibility of conscious life if destroyed. In each case the form of life provides the range of harms that are possible.

These two considerations—health as a primary good and a sensitivity to the ways in which different forms of life can be harmed— narrow but do not determine harm in medicine. Extreme cases are ruled out. A parent who decides that his child does not want to be restored to health can be ignored. A reconstruction of a patient's decision that allows therapeutic pain (suffered, for example, by burn patients) to halt effective treatment is not justified. Within the extremes, however, choices are autonomous. Imagine, for example, a hard case to which probabilties can be assigned. Suppose an individual who, if treated, has a 95 percent chance of being comatose and dependent on a respirator for the rest of his life, and a 5 percent chance of being completely healed. Among the considerations such an individual might survey are the effects of failed treatment on his family and the balance he is prepared to set between unconscious and painful existence versus sentient life. But there is no magic which, when performed, will tell him precisely what he ought to do. A decision that follows the logic of primary goods and is sensitive to the limits and possibilities of life forms is constrained, but offers no axiomatic solution to those cases falling within the constraints.

Notice again that the discretion found in the use of a harm principle is not avoided with rights, and especially not with a right to life. To say that the individual calculating risks against values (positive and negative) is invested with a right to life adds nothing helpful to his decision. To the contrary: a right to life may make decisions less clear. A right to life introduces a final (and high) value for life for all patients that might obscure what a harm principle recognizes—that death may be the most beneficial outcome for some individuals.

A harm principle may be the more basic consideration in life-and-death issues. Maintaining life seems justified on the thought that death harms individuals in the worst possible way. (The opposite logic—justifying a no-harm principle—does not disclose a deeper principle.) But if death can be merciful on occasion, then the principle justifying life may require that death be sought as a way to avoid harm. The best we may be able to do in critical situations within the constraints of primary goods and life forms is to recognize the deeper interests of the individual in avoiding harm. This recognition, painful and imperfect as it often is, reconstructs the conditions of an individual's life to determine how harm can be avoided.

3

The absence of a definition of quality unavoidably grants to staff and parents a wide measure of discretionary authority in therapy decisions in (zone 2) hard cases. This discretion occurs even when decisions are statable in formal terms. Bayesian decision-rules are the most appropriate rules to use in the conditions of uncertainty found in the nursery: here a rational decision combines expected value with probability to yield the best utility return. For example,

the patient trying to decide between a 95 percent chance of unconscious and marginally painful life and a 5 percent chance of full
recovery can try to assign expected value to each of the outcomes.
Say that no treatment leads with certainty to death, which, in the
patient's mind, has a (pragmatic) utility value of -5. Now suppose
that comatose existence is assigned a value of -10 (worse, in the
patient's mind, than death). Intact recovery is given a value of 10.
Then on a calculation of utility,

$$1 (-5) \text{ vs. } .95 (-10) + .05 (10)$$
$$-5 \text{ vs. } -9.5 + .5$$
$$-5 > -9$$

and the patient opts for no treatment.

Or suppose that a variant on Bayesian rules is employed. The von
Neumann-Morgenstern test provides a method for comparing risk
against expected value that gives us a cardinal utility scale unique
for individuals. Imagine that the patient trying to decide on treatment is offered a lottery on an intact life, a, or an unconscious life, b,
in the form of probabilities (p) of a versus b: $p(a) + (1-p) (b)$. This
expression is then compared to the certainty of death, c, by varying
the probabilities (p). A very high probability will incline the patient
to choose therapy; for if the chances are very good that treatment
will be successful, any rational person will decide to be treated. Now
if p is brought slowly down in value, then a point may be reached at
which $p(a) + (1-p)(b) = c$, meaning that the patient is indifferent
between treatment and certain death. (This equilibrium can occur
only if the patient ranks the three alternatives as $a>c>b$, where an
intact life is best but death is preferable to an unconscious life.) A
probability lower than that found at the equilibrium point represents a choice of no treatment and certain death.

Both of these methods can produce rational decisions. But the
rigor of the expressions is misleading. In each of the expressions the
values of life, death, and a permanently comatose state are needed.
In the straightforward Bayesian calculation of expected value
and probability, the values are assigned outright in order to gain
the utility outcomes of each alternative. In the von Neumann-
Morgenstern test the values are disclosed as the probability is
altered. Suppose, however, that one of the alternatives has an
overriding value, one that cannot be set because it is beyond comparing with the alternatives. An intact life would seem to be such a
value. If seen in this way, then patients might select treatment no
matter how low the probability of success on the grounds that an
intact life is worth any risk, no matter what the alternatives are.

A prudent person, however, may find the von Neumann-Morgenstern test a reasonable way to make decisions on therapy. There may well be a point for each of us at which even the best life is equal in value to death when treatment is highly likely to produce a permanent comatose condition. But the utility scale so disclosed is *unique* to each individual. The point of equilibrium for one patient need not be the point for any other. Nor are there any tests that will say one point is more rational than another. Each patient has the discretionary authority to set the point where he wishes. The reason for this is that the values of the alternatives are open, not closed by any system of value.

This discretionary zone for decisions is set more firmly in place by the open-textured quality of the main normative concepts in medicine. "Human being," for example, is a term with both biological and evaluative senses. A biological indicator of humanness exists. All members of the human species have forty-six chromosomes of a distinctive type. But the biological markets of species do not lead to any evaluative claims. Evaluative languages—especially those of rights—are focused on human characteristics that are not restricted to species. Sentience, for example, is a common condition underlying a variety of rights (including, on some arguments, the right to life). Sentience, however, extends to higher vertebrates who do not have human biological markers. The use of the term "human being" to direct or guide decisions on treatment is bound, therefore, to fail. There is nothing unique about human beings that prescribes a course of treatment limited to humans. Decisions using a definition of humanness as a guide are at the discretion of the decision maker.

Even "interests" remain open. Stephanie Christopher lived in great pain for the entire duration of her brief life. Suppose that physicians were guided by Stephanie's best interests. Did they follow their own guidelines in deciding whether and how to treat her? Even looking back on the treatment, with the advantage of hindsight, it is difficult to say. On an interpretation of interests that is restricted to a narrow egoism, Stephanie would probably have been better off if she had died quickly without having to endure pain. But interests can extend to others. The travail of Stephanie's life touched many people deeply. Her parents are different people now, transformed by the experience. Others see the world in different ways as a result of knowing Stephanie. It is conceivable that a Stephanie who knew the full implication of those effects would have chosen to live the way she did live for nine weeks and part of a day. Her interests might have extended to all of those around her. The problem is that we cannot say. A rational, competent Stephanie is a part of our imagination, and as part of our imagination we can construct her choices as we wish. We *choose* her best interests. We do not discover them.

The main normative concepts in medicine are not precisely defined. There are multiple standards for their correct use, and these standards represent different communities of value. Neither rational argument nor appeals to evidence can resolve disputes over their uses. There are, as a consequence, always good reasons to support one or another of the interpretations of the concepts. It is not mysterious, seen in this way, that the alternative choices on therapy can often *all* be reasonable depending on your point of view; for the concepts that defend and justify the alternatives admit of contrary but equally appealing interpretations. Both "humanness" and "best interest," for example, can lead consistently to opposed courses of treatment—depending on how they are interpreted.

4

Medical practice in neonatology has a normative structure. There are precise and indisputable rules and procedures. The principles of care are settled. Some of this structure is found in all rational inquiry. Physicians generalize from data, use evidence in imaginative ways to diagnose problems, employ theoretical principles, and accept critical reflections on their work from colleagues. So too do scientists, gamblers, and other rational practitioners. Other features of medicine help mark off medical practices from some, though not all, rational inquiries. Physicians stress the importance of particular cases (as opposed to the generalities celebrated in empirical science). The reciprocal effects between facts and theories seem particularly strong in medicine. Doctors look at cases and allow their observations to modify theories. This essentially inductive method, though informed by clinical experience and theory, contrasts markedly with deductive forms of explanation (where conclusions are derived from subsuming particular events under universal laws). We have also seen how medicine is remedial, incremental, and dependent on cooperation among staff colleagues.

This normative structure is not discretionary. A doctor who presumes individual authority over the rules and procedures of medicine will encounter resistance from other practitioners. But within the structure, and even because of the structure, those deciding on therapy seem always to have a measure of discretion. Knowledge in medicine is incomplete and interpretable (to some degree) from a variety of perspectives. It is in part for this reason that skill seems to be as important as knowledge (or even experience) in medical therapy. Nurses correctly see that good doctors are not always those who are most familiar with the latest research. A good doctor is contextually good, good in a particular relationship to her patient. Doctoring seems to be a type of good judgment that, while requiring a base of knowledge, is not deduced in any axiomatic way from the base of knowledge. Even the virtues embedded in medicine reflect the open quality of therapy decisions. Useful virtues in medicine include honesty, tolerance, openness, a capacity to employ fair arguments and use facts honestly, a willingness to compromise. All of these virtues complement a rational system in which value is created by individuals who have the autonomy to make decisions. They are inconsistent with a rational system that closes out individual discretion on authoritative grounds.

The open quality of therapy decisions is precisely what makes medical practice a fertile ground of community conflicts over therapy. The goals of *life* and *health* in medicine can be weighted in different ways from a variety of perspectives. A viable life from certain religious perspectives may be any life in any form. Those who embrace a doctrine of life's sanctity under all conditions introduce to medicine a community of value that can set life against health; for some patients can be restored to life even when it is impossible to restore their health. A viable life to most doctors means survival at a certain minimal level of health, including a reasonably functioning neurological system. But each interpretation of life, and even of health, is coherent within the contrasting communities of religion and medicine. That therapy decisions have such open-ended goals makes contests over their meaning particularly appropriate in medical practice.

The lesson so clearly expressed by the logic of therapy decisions is that ambiguity is built into the decisions. There can always be disputes over therapy because discretion is a logical feature of therapy decisions. As with paradigms that are incommensurable, the disputants may not always share a common language. But the competing points of view are rational in terms of the community values from which they derive. Given the disputable character of values in therapy decisions, the instruments to make decisions must disclose possible equilibrium points on which the parties can agree. The mechanisms of negotiation and compromise among parents and doctors seem appropriate for this task. The legal system does not.

The political community is unlike other communities in its capacity to adjudicate and order the claims of communities. Politics is the process of doing this when there are no overriding criteria to say which of the competing communities is right and which wrong. It is the performance of this external function that requires the use of fairness and proportionality, criteria of sameness and difference, perhaps utility, in just governing. Distance and impersonality are needed to rank values that cannot be ranked on tests internal to communities. Special commitments, like those nutured in friendships, might be the dominant influence in decisions made within communities. Prudential or practical wisdoms may guide decisions among those loyal to particular values. But the political community is bound by more objective principles.

One issue in pluralist societies is the relationship between the political community and other communities. In the neonatal nursery, the issue takes the form of this question: Are the interests of infants best recognized through negotiations among communities, or by the legal instruments of the political community? Among the considerations in answering this question are (a) what internal changes are required in a community as a result of a political resolution, and (b) the relative ease of internal accommodations and self-regulation (as with the use of Infant Care Review Committees). The rational pattern of therapy decisions suggests that the interests of infants are best determined from within medical practices by doctors and parents. One reason for this is that these interests seem to be a particular amalgam of life and health that is disclosed by discussion between doctors and parents. The amalgam does not exist prior to the discussion.

The importance of community values also diminishes the relevance of rights in therapy decisions. Rights do not clarify, and sometimes obfuscate, the interests of babies in the nursery. A right to life ignores the fact that *health* is the primary goal of medicine, not simply the maintenance of life. A right is a blocking device, a term that sets the individual off from the community. What is needed in neonatal nurseries is a clear statement on how individual interests occur within communities. Also, the extension of rights to life to forms of life distant from ideals of autonomy and sentience distorts the use of rights language. The confusions and anomalies of therapy decisions seem to arise in part as we ask the language of rights to do more than it can do. In extending rights languages to such life forms we are forced to maintain that these forms are identical to sovereign individuals in all moral respects. The strangeness of this claim can be seen immediately when it is maintained, for example, that anencephalic babies have the same right to life as sentient and rational adults because the two forms of life are morally identical.

Finally, an expanded concept of *harm* seems to be a more effective device to identify the interests of infants. There is no use pretending that the harm concept can provide principles that will transform therapy decisions from an interpretive to a precise science. The representatives of children will still have wide discretionary authority with the use of harm as a guide to interests. But the medical community does provide reasonable limits to discretion. The primary good of *health* constrains decisions by stating the purpose of medical therapy and identifying the interests of patients in the nursery. But those interests are notoriously difficult to fix in hard cases. Worse: the presence of competing communities in the nursery introduces different schedules of interests. Nothing is currently available to rank those communities, nor will be available so long as individuals are the focus of value in society (no matter how sensitive such values are to community perspectives). A reconstruction of harm is at least sensitive to differences among communities.

The problem in therapy decisions in neonatal nurseries is how to act rationally on behalf of infants. This study provides a sketch of what such representational rationality ought to look like in neonatalogy. Decisions should (a) be the products of negotiations between doctors and parents, (b) make little or no reference to rights, and (c) use harm as a constraint on decisions. To decide on the basis of more objective rules and values would require that individuals be seen as independent of communities. And then therapy in hard cases would often make no sense whatsoever.

5

May 11. In nursery briefly this morning. Jay O'Brien sees me in the hall and asks if I want to attend an autopsy. Stephanie's. I answer yes. We go downstairs together to the morgue in the subbasement of the hospital. It is a very cold place. The pathologist conducting the autopsy looks like a friendly neighborhood butcher. He is fat with a heavy mustache and wears a white gown that looks like an apron. I pass myself off as a physician, even managing (to O'Brien's bemusement) to answer a few questions on Stephanie's treatment.

Stephanie's body is on a table. She is opened up, a cadaver now.

People can do whatever they need to do with what remains of her. She looks exactly like a stiff doll and not at all human any longer. Her face, in the repose of death, seems unmarked. One can imagine her in a hypothetical future, not to be realized, as a sleepy-eyed teenager with long hair.

At moments like this it is eminently clear that we live as individuals in and through a limited range of physical conditions. These conditions provide us with our identities. Death is the breakdown of these conditions. The physical basis of life is nowhere more clearly expressed than in an autopsy. The anomaly of Stephanie's life is that she fought against her physical endowments. She lived a contradiction. If all human effort forms a normative grid of existence, then Stephanie's efforts are somewhere on this grid. I wish I could locate them to make sense of her life.

Upstairs, in the level 2 wing of the nursery, the room in which Stephanie lived and died is empty. No air circulates in the room at this moment. No one is present.

A resident sits down on a bench with me in the hall outside what was Stephanie's room. She is in a reflective mood. "Children," she tells me, "always get a longer code than adults. People around here feel that the death of a child is the worst thing. They do everything to save them. The parents are here. The children are so young. But I've seen old people die alone, with no one there. To me, that's the worst thing. To die alone when you're old."

I wonder.

> *From the interview with Mr. and Mrs. Raymond. Danielle has woken up from her nap, and Mrs. Raymond has brought her downstairs, where I hold her. Danielle seems to be making a complete recovery from her early and almost fatal beginnings. She is very pretty and does not look at all like the diminutive infant I saw in the nursery.*

Frohock: She's beautiful. She really looks different.

Mr. Raymond: Yes, she's gotten better.

Frohock: How much does she weigh now?

Mrs. Raymond: She's up to eleven pounds and the doctors are proud of her.

Frohock: And she's alert, no problems?

Mr. Raymond: No problems at all. She's very alert.

Frohock: How did Danielle look when you first saw her?

Mr. Raymond: Well, she was real small, real skinny. I'd say she wasn't more than about two inches across, it looked like to me, and she was only thirteen inches long or smaller than that. She didn't look human. She looked like a little monkey or something because of all the hair and the way her eyes were sunken way back in her head. And her fingers—it looked like there was hardly any skin on them at all. When I saw her heart beat, I saw it push the skin away and right there I just couldn't stay there any more. I had to leave.

Frohock: When did she start looking human to you?

Mr. Raymond: I don't know how long before she started looking human to my wife, but I took them down [to Northeastern] about five or six times before I'd ever go in again. And it was about that time when I went in again that she looked like a normal baby. She'd gotten more color to her. She was more white and, I don't know, she just looked better to me.

Frohock: How about you?

Mrs. Raymond: Well, just like he says, she was—they said that she seemed more alert. When she cried, she cried like a baby lamb would cry. That's the way she would cry.

Frohock: Let me ask you a question. It may seem strange looking at this gorgeous child, but suppose the doctors had told you that she would not be at all normal. Would you have said no on treatment?

Mr. Raymond: No. I don't care if she—right now, they can't tell until she's a year old whether she had any brain damage. But I don't really care. She's made it this far. She's going to make it the rest of the way as far as I'm concerned. There's nothing going to hold her back. Nothing to hold me back from loving her as much either. Even if she does turn out to be mentally retarded. The way she is now, as alert as she is—she looks around at everything. You can call her name and she'll look right at you. She's alert and she's got good eye contact and good reflexes. So I don't think anything's going to be wrong with her. I think she's going to be a normal healthy baby now.

Frohock: So then we're really, I guess, looking back on easy decisions?

Mr. Raymond: Well, the first one was tough.

Frohock: What made it tough?

Mr. Raymond: Well, just thinking about it afterwards was the hardest thing for me. Because right then I was worried the whole time until I got to see her. I didn't know whether she was going to make it on the ride to Northeastern or if she was going to make it anywhere. She was on oxygen the whole time. They said they had tubes running in and out of her and that she weighed 1 pound. Well, they told me she weighed one pound, five ounces, and that had me scared right there because she was so small. But, like I said, I made the decision and I wanted her to be with us. I wanted her to live.

Frohock: In general, do you think the quality of a child's life ought to be a factor in making decisions on treatment?

Mr. Raymond: I don't think you should consider it because most people when they have kids nowadays, they plan on having them. So, if you plan on having one, you might as well take what the Lord gives you. Because it's up to Him whether or not the baby's going to be mentally retarded or if it's going to be disabled or anything. I figure nowadays when you're going to have a kid, you're taking a 50/50 chance whether or not it's going to be normal or if it's going to be abnormal. But there's no reason, even if it's abnormal, not to love it like it was a normal baby. Because it's your kid—it's your daughter or your son.

Frohock: So they should always treat, under all circumstances?

Mr. Raymond: Right. They should just treat them all the same, I think.

From the interview with Stephanie's parents

Mrs. Christopher: We went to genetic counseling in Northeastern and we went through our family trees. They told us that in order for the baby to have this skin disease, both my husband and I had to be carriers of it. They told us that if I was to get pregnant again, there would be a 75 percent chance that it wouldn't happen again, but a 25 percent chance that it would. So I decided that I'd wait and see. Well, then we talked it over and we decided that we'd try to have another baby. I got pregnant and they told me that when I was twenty-two to twenty-three weeks along, that I'd go to New Haven, Connecticut, and have a fetoscopy test done. This is where they stick a needle or something down through my stomach to the baby and take skin grafts to tell whether or not the baby had the disease.

We had to take a bus all the way down and all the way back. The night that we got home my water broke. I went to the hospital and that stopped for a while—a week. I went home for one day. Then I went back to the hospital because I started leaking fluid again. They told me that I'd lose the baby because of the fluid that I was putting out. Then I stopped leaking again. The time that I was in the hospital here in Allenville they told me—well, they called from New Haven and they told me that from the test results they couldn't tell anything except that the baby was a girl and that she had O positive blood. So they told me that I had a choice. Either come back and have the test done again or just hope that nothing happens that I lose the baby. So we went through with the pregnancy. I was here in Allenville for three weeks and then I started leaking a lot of blood. They sent me to Northeastern. I was down there from February 2d to March 10th, when I delivered the baby. I was only thirty weeks along. She weighed two pounds, eleven ounces, which is small.

During the time that I was in the hospital, Bill was running back and forth from Allenville to Northeastern. They were giving me shots to develop the baby's lungs. In case I did deliver early, her lungs would hopefully be developed enough where she could breathe on her own and not have to worry about it. They were also giving me shots for cramps— premature labor or whatever they want to call it—and they'd give me a shot and it'd go away. Then the last time, they gave me a shot and it didn't work and I just delivered the baby. I started having cramps around 4:00 in the afternoon and 11:44 that night I delivered. When she was born she had a small spot here on her nose where the skin had come off. It was indented. She also had a patch of skin on the top of her hand that had started to come off. They weren't sure then if the baby had the skin disease or not. I didn't want to believe that, because I'd already gone through it once before and I didn't want to go through it again. While I was down in the recovery room, I called up to the third floor to see how she was doing. They said, "Well, she's doing fine. She's got a little bit of skin coming off her stomach." And I still didn't want to believe it.

Finally when I did get a chance to go up to see her, the first thing I asked them was if they put tape on her. The nurse told me that they did and she said "Well, we took it off." I said, "When you did that, did the skin come off with it?" She said "Yes." I knew right then that she had it because with the disease, you can't put anything on the skin. You can't put any pressure on the skin. If you do this to them, the skin would just shear right off. It was almost like their mind was telling them that they didn't need their skin—to just get rid of it. So I told the nurse not to pick her up if they didn't have to. Only if it was absolutely necessary pick her up, and not to put any more tape on her, because it'd only take her skin off with it. So they put a sign on her bed saying minimum handling and no tape. First they had her in an isolette and then they sent to Nashville, Tennessee, for this special bed—the one that you probably saw her in.

January 13. Sunday. The annual party for alumni of the special care nursery is being held today in the hospital cafeteria. A special room has been decorated at the back of the main hall. Streamers hang down from the ceiling with blue and red and pink balloons attached. A large table against the back wall offers guests generous helpings of cheese and crackers, fresh broccoli, carrots, celery. Trays of brownies and chocolate cake surround a punch bowl filled with a pink mixture of Hawaiian Punch.

At the entrance to the room is a large sign: "Welcome Neonate Nursery Alumni—Please Sign In and Leave a Mailing Address." Two nurses are supervising an informal registration of parents. Soon the room is filled with families talking to one another. The parents compare lengths of stay. "Kevin was in the nursery for seventy-one days," one mother tells another. Illnesses are dissected clinically. "Brian weighed one pound, six ounces, when he was admitted. He had two bad bleeds. Can you believe it? Look at him now." Brian, the object of this reference, is trying to unhook the fire extinguisher from the wall. "Mary had NEC. They gave up on her. I can remember when five grams of formula was a victory. Now she can't stop eating." Mary is a chubby baby asleep on her mother's shoulder.

Some of the special care nurses are moving about the room, shrieking with delight when they come upon a child who was special to them. Mary Jane Kennedy is out of uniform, off duty, dressed in plaid slacks, fashion boots, a black and white sweater blouse, her hair pulled back and down to her waist in back. "You kept your hair," one mother tells her. "I'll never cut this hair," she responds. She sits down next to a little girl who is eating ice cream. "Do you remember me?" The girl turns to Kennedy and opens her arms wide. Kennedy picks her up with a broad smile. "You are a sweetheart," she tells the girl.

Soon the room is filled and families are occupying tables in the main cafeteria room. Many of the children are running from one table to another. Some show the ravages of disease and treatment. A few are limping. Some mouths and noses are off center. Several children have the large and protruding eyes that sometimes follow extensive time on a ventilator. Others are wearing thick glasses. But on the whole the scene is filled with happy and noisy children who appear normal. The parents are eating, gossiping, trying to keep track of their broods.

A mother holding a baby has cornered Kennedy. "He's still not nursing. But he eats tremendously," she tells Kennedy. "You know the pediatrician asked me last month if I was looking at my child through a microscope. I said, 'Sure. Wouldn't you?'"

Kennedy laughs. "At least you don't own a stethoscope."

The woman shrugs. "What would I listen for? What do I know about the heart?" She moves closer. "But I do measure his head still. The last thing I did was steal a bunch of those tapes to measure head circumference." The woman grabs Kennedy's arm and they laugh together.

The woman's child is growing. His head is getting bigger. She is happy in her preoccupations. Missing from this party are the parents of children who did not survive the special care nursery, or who have simply decided to skip the party. Michael Anthony died last October. Stephanie Christopher's parents are at home in their trailer this afternoon with their son. Jill Monihan still sleeps upstairs in pediatrics (the debate continuing over whether she is indeed a survivor). Cindy Blackwell is in Chicago being treated for neurological problems. Warren Carr has died. Danielle Raymond is playing at home with her brother. Jill Simon is just waking up from her nap to be held and fed by her parents in a large, comfortable house.

The party is now dense with parents and their children. It is a happy scene. No ghosts are here today. The memories of the special care nursery are mediated and transformed by the survival of the children. A visitor coming upon this celebration would never guess by looking at the families what some of them have experienced.

Glossary

The definitions below come from *Taber's Cyclopedic Medical Dictionary*, 14th edition, ed. by Clayton L. Thomas (Philadelphia: F.A. Davis Co., 1982); *Manual of Neonatal Care*, ed. by John P. Cloherty, M.D., and Ann R. Stark, M.D. (Boston: Little, Brown, & Co., 1983); Henry K. Silver, C. Henry Kempe, and Henry B. Bruyn, *Handbook of Pediatrics*, 14th edition (Los Altos, California: Lange Medical Publications, 1983); and from consultations with physicians and nurses. I have not included well-known terms, medications, or terms used once with a definition appended in the text.

anencephalus. Congenital absence of brain and (sometimes) spinal cord.

Apgar. System to score an infant's physical condition immediately after birth. Five objective signs—heart rate, respiration, muscle tone, response to stimuli, and color—are each given a score of 0, 1, or 2. A total score of 10 indicates an infant in perfect physical condition.

apnea. Temporary cessation of breathing.

beta strep. Beta-hemolytic streptococcal infections. A disease of newborn infants caused by group B streptococci.

CAT. Computerized axial tomography. A method of securing anatomical information about the body by using X-rays and computer-generated images.

colostomy. The opening of some portion of the colon onto the abdominal wall. Performed surgically when feces cannot pass through the colon and out of the anus.

CPAP. Continuous positive airway pressure. A device that supplies air under pressure through a mask, nasal prongs, or a tube.

CPR. Cardiopulmonary resuscitation.

cyanosis. A deficiency of oxygen in the blood that causes a bluish or slatelike appearance of the skin.

EEG. Electroencephalogram. A tracing of electrical activity in the brain.

hyaline membrane disease. A disease of the lungs of newborn infants which prevents the baby from receiving an adequate supply of oxygen through unaided breathing.

hydrocephalus. Increased accumulation of cerebrospinal fluid within the ventricles of the brain.

hypoplastic left heart. Defective development of the left side of the heart.

I.V. Intravenous. Any device used to introduce medication, fluids, or nutrients directly into a vein of a patient.

NEC. Necrotizing enterocolitis. A severe, often fatal disease of the intestines that occurs predominantly in low-birth-weight preterm infants. The cause of the disease is unknown.

PFC. Persistant fetal circulation. Conditions in which pulmonary artery hypertension prevents a successful transition from fetal to extrauterine circulatory patterns. In effect, the infant remains in the circulatory patterns of a fetus after birth.

PCO$_2$. Carbon dioxide level in the blood.

pH factor. Potential of hydrogen. A measure of the degree of acidity or alkalinity of blood (or any substance). The normal pH of blood is 7.4.

PO$_2$. Oxygen level in the blood.

sepsis. Infection in the blood stream due to the presence of microorganisms or their poisonous products.

serum electrolytes. Chemicals (sodium, chloride, potassium, bicarbonate, etc.) found in the fluid portion of the blood (that portion of the blood that remains after the removal of the fibrin clot and the blood cells). Often used to designate a balance or concentration of these ions in the body.

spina bifida. Congenital defect in walls of the spinal canal caused by lack of union between the layers of the vertebrae. It occurs about once in 1,000 live births.

trisomy 13. An extra (third) chromosome of the 13th pair. Severe congenital deformation and mental retardation result. Children with the condition usually do not survive past the first year of life.

trisomy 18. An extra (third) chromosome of the 18th pair. It causes severe deformity and mental retardation. Survival past the first year of life is unusual.

trisomy 21. Down's syndrome. The extra chromosome (of the 21st pair) causes mental retardation and physical deformity. The condition occurs in one of every 700 live births.

ventilator/respirator. A mechanical device for artificial ventilation of the lungs.

Bibliography

Since the primary goal of *Special Care* is to reconstruct the ordinary life of a neonatal nursery, it is understandable that the views of participants in medical practice guide the work. But, in addition to describing how practitioners see ethical and other problems, I have introduced at various points in the narrative some reflections on the issues and problems of neonatal intensive care. The research material I found especially helpful in forming my reflections is listed below with comments on each item. This annotated bibliography should be a resource for the reader wishing to go beyond the account of neonatology offered here.

Let me first mention the works that inform and justify the ethnographic approach I use. Especially helpful, on the techniques of interviewing, is James P. Spradley's *The Ethnographic Interview* (New York: Holt, Rinehart & Winston, 1979). The philosophies of social inquiry endorsed here are developed in Alfred Schutz, *Collected Papers*, 3 volumes, edited by Maurice Natanson (The Hague: Martinus Nijhoff, 1967); Clifford Geertz, *The Interpretation of Cultures* (New York: Basic Books, 1973)—though I give different interpretations here, I think, to the notion of "thick description"; Ludwig Wittgenstein, *Philosophical Investigations* (New York: Macmillan, 1953); John Searle, *Speech Acts* (Cambridge: Cambridge University Press, 1969); Michel Foucault, *The Order of Things: An Archeology of the Human Sciences* (New York: Pantheon, 1971); Alasdair MacIntyre, *A Short History of Ethics* (New York: Macmillan, 1966) and *After Virtue* (Notre Dame, Ind.: University of Notre Dame Press, 1981); and, in spite of the author's recent decline in importance, R. G. Collingwood, *The Idea of History* (New York: Oxford, 1956). This list could be expanded ad infinitum (or so it seems to me at times). But in these seminal works, different though they are from one another in style and content, can be found the elaborations of a rule-following, intentional, basically *internal* side to social practices that I try to describe here in this case study of neonatology.

1. Neonatology: Diseases, Nursing, Statistics, Case Histories

The medical literature is important in establishing base lines with which to understand and assess the practices of the neonatal nursery. I have in-

227

cluded a number of articles I found especially helpful in learning about Stephanie Christopher's fatal illness.

Adashi, Eli Y., Farid J. Louis, and Maria Vasquez. "An Unusual Case of Epidermolysis Bullosa Hereditaria Letalis with Cutaneous Scarring and Pyloric Atresia." *Journal of Pediatrics* 96 (March 1980): 443–46.

   This article reports on a rare case of epidermolysis bullosa letalis in which the patient suffered serious scarring. Pyloric atresia, a constriction of the stomach outlet sometimes associated with epidermolysis bullosa letalis, was also present.

Anton-Lamprecht, Ingrun. "Genetically Induced Abnormalities of Epidermal Differentiation and Ultrastructure in Ichthyoses and Epidermolysis: Pathogenisis, Heterogeneity, Fetal Manifestation and Prenatal Diagnosis." *Journal of Investigative Dermatology* 81 (1983): 1949–56.

   An examination of certain genetic interactions during developmental processes. The relationship between mutant genes and the diseases listed in the title of the article serves as a focus for the work.

Brans, Yves W., and others. "Perinatal Mortality in a Large Perinatal Center: Five Year Review of 31,000 Births." *American Journal of Obstetrics and Gynecology* 148 (February 1984): 284–89.

   The authors provide statistics on the causes of death at a special care facility and also detail causes of death and mortality rates for infants of different birth weights.

Budetti, Peter P., and Peggy McManus. "Assessing the Effectiveness of Neonatal Intensive Care." *Medical Care* 20 (October 1982): 1027–39.

   The authors collect and analyze data available from studies of isolated intensive care units. By pooling the data and recalculating statistics they conclude that neonatal intensive care units have significantly reduced infant mortality in the United States since 1965.

Ciba Foundation. *Major Mental Handicap: Methods and Costs of Prevention.* New York: Elsevier, Excerpta Medica, North Holland, 1978.

   These papers, first presented at a Ciba Foundation Symposium, range from cost-benefit analysis on preventing mental handicaps, to methods for evaluating newborns, to results of studies on the causes of mental handicaps in infants.

David, Richard J., and Earl Siegel. "Decline in Neonatal Mortality, 1968–1977: Better Babies or Better Care?" *Pediatrics* 71 (April 1983): 531–40.

   A study of births over a decade demonstrates that there has been a significant trend toward higher birth weights and longer gestations. This trend can, in part, account for lower mortality rates. The authors also recognize significant decreases in mortality at given birth weights. These decreases support the thought that special care nurseries have been successful in reducing infant mortality.

Desmond, Murdina M., and others. "The Very Low Birth Weight Infant after Discharge from Intensive Care: Anticipatory Health Care and Developmental Course." *Current Problems in Pediatrics* April 1980, 1–59.

Studies on the long-term effect of prematurity suggest (without conclusive evidence) that premature children are "at risk" at least through school age. The authors urge parents and pediatricians to an early diagnosis of problems that may affect a child later in life. Suggestions for behavioral management and education are also offered.

El Shafie, M., and others. "Pyloric Atresia and Epidermolysis Bullosa Letalis: A Lethal Combination in Two Premature Newborn Siblings." *Journal of Pediatric Surgery* 14 (August 1979): 446–49.

The case histories described in this paper suggest a linkage between two genetic diseases—pyloric atresia and epidermolysis bullosa letalis.

Elwood, J. Mark, and J. Harold Elwood. *Epidemiology of Anencephalus and Spina Bifida.* Oxford: Oxford University Press, 1980.

This study relates two of the most common congenital defects to various environmental and genetic factors. The authors also discuss prenatal diagnosis and the legal and ethical questions which surround defective fetuses. Their analysis includes a study of cases and law from both the United Kingdom and the United States.

Gortmaker, S., and others. "The Survival of Very Low Birth-Weight Infants by Level of Hospital of Birth: A Papulation Study of Perinatal Systems in Four States." *American Journal of Obstetrics and Gynecology* 152, no. 5 (July 1, 1985): 517–24.

This study indicates that very low birth-weight infants born at high technology centers have better odds of survival than those born at regular urban or rural hospitals. The results underscore the importance of neonatal intensive care units in reducing infant mortality.

Heredia-Perez, J. A. "A Special Care Baby." *Nursing Times* 76 (May 1, 1980), 778–82.

A case study of a premature baby treated in a special care nursery. Details of vital statistics such as weight and feeding regimen are also provided.

Holmes, Deborah L., Jill Nagy Reich, and Joseph F. Pasternak. *The Development of Infants Born at Risk.* Hillside, N.J.: Lawrence Erlbaum Assoc. Publishers, 1984.

This text documents all aspects of development in newborns born at risk, from birth and activities in special care nurseries to the possible long-term effects of the disabilities experienced by high-risk infants.

Kerr, Kathleen. "Reporting the Case of Baby Jane Doe." *Hastings Center Report* 14 (August 1984): 7–9.
    The public history of the Baby Jane Doe case, including the federal government's response to the case.

Klaus, Marshall, and John Kennell. "Interventions in the Premature Nursery: Impact on Development." *Pediatric Clinics of North America* 29 (October 1982): 1263–73.
    The authors discuss several studies on mother-child contact following premature births. They suggest methods that nurseries can use to enhance these contacts. The contacts can foster healthy bonding between parent and child and relieve guilt that the mother often feels following a premature birth.

Korones, Sheldon B. *High Risk Newborn Infant: The Basis for Intensive Nursing Care.* 3d ed. St. Louis: C. V. Mosby Co., 1981.
    This nursing text discusses most aspects of neonatal care. Included are sections on the organization of special care nurseries, the significance of birth weight, lung disorders, hemotologic disorders, infection, defects of the central nervous system, and the effect of neonatal intensive care on parent-child relations.

McLaughlin, John F., David B. Shurtleff, Janice Y. Lamers, J. Timothy Stuntz, Patricia W. Hayden, and Robert J. Kropp. "Influence of Prognosis on Decisions Regarding the Care of Newborns with Myelodysplasia." *New England Journal of Medicine* 312 (June 20, 1985): 1589–94.
    Using criteria from their earlier study, the authors conclude that early surgical care is now increasing survival rates among infants with spina bifida disorders. Survival has not improved for those infants receiving only supportive care.

Meier, Paula Primmer. "A Crisis Group for Parents of High-Risk Infants." *Maternal-Child Nursing Journal* 7 (Spring 1978): 21–30.
    The author describes the formation and use of group therapy to provide counseling for parents of infants in a special care nursery. Recurring themes in counseling help illuminate the problems that parents have in coping with high-risk infants.

Milligan, J. E., A. T. Shennan, and E. M. Hoskins. "Perinatal Intensive Care: Where and How to Draw the Line." *American Journal of Obstetrics and Gynecology* 148 (March 1984): 499–503.
    The authors use clinical data in an attempt to demonstrate the probability of survival for low birth-weight infants. They suggest

that the possibility of survival is restricted for infants born at or below a gestational age of twenty-five weeks.

Peltier, Frank A., Eduardo H. Tschen, Sharon S. Raimer, and Tseng-tong Kus. "Epidermolysis Bullosa Letalis Associated with Congenital Pyloric Atresia." *Archives of Dermatology* 117 (November 1981): 728–31.

A case study and subsequent review of other case histories reveal an association between the presence of epidermolysis bullosa letalis and congenital pyloric atresia, a constriction at the outlet of the stomach.

Poland, R. L., and others. "Analysis of the Effects of Applying Federal Diagnosis-Related Grouping Guidelines to a Population of High Risk Newborn Infants." *Pediatrics* 76, no. 1 (July 1985): 104–9.

The authors claim serious discrepancies between federal estimates of time needed for tertiary care in hospitals and the actual length of time needed for this care. This suggests that implementation of the federal system of DRGs and consequent payments would severely discourage tertiary care referral hospitals from providing intensive neonatal care.

Rebone, Joseph W. " 'Minimal Quality of Life': Why Parents, Courts Chose Infant Doe's Death." *Hospital Progress* 14 (June 1982): 10–12, 14.

A member of the Indiana Right to Life organization tells the story of infant Doe and of the association's efforts to get a favorable court ruling on the parents' and doctors' responsibilities to the child.

Rodeck, C. H., R. A. J. Eady, and C. M. Goshen. "Prenatal Diagnosis of Epidermolysis Bullosa Letalis." *The Lancet*, May 3, 1980, 949–952.

The authors report success in diagnosing this skin disease in a fetus at eighteen weeks' gestation.

Ross, G., and others. "Physical Growth and Developmental Outcome in Very Low Birth Weight Premature Infants at Three Years of Age." *Journal of Pediatrics* 107, no. 2 (August 1985): 284–89.

An assessment of low birth-weight infants at three years of age shows that these infants remain smaller and have poor neurological functioning as compared to infants of normal term and weight.

Rudolph, Abraham M., and Julian I. E. Hoffmoan. *Pediatrics.* Connecticut: Appleton-Century Crofts, 1982.

A general textbook on pediatric medicine.

Santulli, Thomas V. "Acute Necrotizing Enterocolitis: Recognition and Management." *Hospital Practice* 9 (November 1974): 129–35.

Clinical testing that suggests a possible treatment for this disease is reported in this article. Santulli also claims that breastfeeding can compensate for deficiencies in the immunologic systems of high-risk infants.

Schachner, Lawrence, Gerald S. Lazarus, and Herbert Dembitzer. "Epidermolysis Bullosa Hereditaria Letalis: Pathology, Natural History and Therapy." *British Journal of Dermatology* 96 (1977): 51–58.
    This article reports on a treatment that resulted in a significant reduction in blistering by the patient.

Sheldon, Robert E., ed. *The Expanding Role of the Nurse in Neonatal Intensive Care.* New York: Grune & Stratton, 1980.
    This text includes articles on the legal status of nurses, the nurse's role as seen by physicians, the selection of nurses for special care nurseries, and other topics.

Smith, Janis Bloedel, ed. *Pediatric Critical Care.* New York: John Wiley & Sons, 1983.
    The reader will find a summary of the diseases and defects likely to be encountered in special care nursing. The volume documents symptoms and treatments for the common medical problems nurses will encounter.

Sondheimer, Henry M., Craig J. Byrum, and Marie S. Blackman. "Unequal Cardiac Care for Children with Down's Syndrome." *American Journal of Diseases in Children* 139 (January 1985): 68–71.
    This study concludes that Down's Syndrome children suffering from congenital complete artrioventricular canal defect can be successfully treated if the referral comes at an early age. As the child ages, the condition cannot be treated due to the progressive nature of the defect. Late referral denies such patients the benefits of standard cardiac care.

Stinson, Robert, and Peggy Stinson. *The Long Dying of Baby Andrew.* Boston: Little, Brown & Co., 1983.
    The daily journals kept by the Stinsons through the short life of their child describe personal emotional struggles as well as struggles with the hospital bureaucracy as their premature baby was treated with all available resources—treatment which merely delayed his inevitable death.

Wallis, Sheila and D. Harvey. "Respiratory Distress: Its Cause and Management." *Nursing Times* 75 (July 26, 1979): 1264–72.
    Common respiratory illnesses in newborns are reviewed in this article. The authors also detail methods for mechanically assisting respiration, the use of physiotherapy and blood gases, and techniques for weaning infants from respirators.

2. Legal Analysis and Legal Cases

The relations between law and neonatal medicine are explored in a number of ways in the relevant literature. I have listed here the articles I found most helpful in the area of therapy decisions on infant children. Two qualifications must be stated. First, some of the references in this section overlap with the moral and philosophical themes of section 4. This is to be expected, given the moral controversies over law in these areas. Second, I have not listed an important area of legal scholarship treating the limitations of law as an instrument of conflict resolution or management. The best general resource in this area is probably Donald Horowitz, *The Courts and Social Policy* (Washington, D.C.: The Brookings Institution, 1977). See also the discussion of law and community by Jerold S. Auerbach, *Justice without Law?* (Oxford: Oxford University Press, 1983).

American Academy of Pediatrics. "A Proposal for an Ethics Committee." *Hastings Center Report* 13 (December 1983): 6–7.

The American Academy of Pediatrics submitted this proposal in response to the U.S. Department of Health and Human Services' call for comments on its proposed regulations.

Annas, George J. "'A Wonderful Case and an Irrational Tragedy': The Philip Becker Case Continues." *Hastings Center Report* 12 (February 1982): 25–26.

Two court cases are discussed, involving Philip Becker's parent's attempts to avoid corrective heart surgery and the attempts of some "psychological parents" to obtain guardian status and provide Becker with the surgery.

———. "Defining Death: There Ought to Be a Law." *Hastings Center Report* 13 (February 1983): 20–21.

Annas discusses the Uniform Determination of Death Act and explains the legal and policy reasons for such an act.

———. "Disconnecting the Baby Doe Hotline." *Hastings Center Report* 13 (June 1983), 14–16.

A description of the Department of Health and Human Services' first attempt at protecting handicapped newborns through administrative regulation. The rules fell before litigation that challenged the procedures used by HHS in adopting them.

———. "Baby Doe Redux: Doctors as Child Abusers." *Hastings Center Report* 13 (October 1983): 26–27.

Annas reviews the development and the content of the final regulations issued by the Department of Health and Human Services following the Baby Jane Doe case.

Auerbach, Jerold S. *Justice without Law?* Oxford: Oxford University Press, 1983.

A discussion of the ways in which law expresses individualism and an exploration of the natural tensions between litigiousness and the communitarian visions that give meaning to individual lives.

Baumgardner, Karl Leland. "Defective Newborns: Inconsistent Application of Legal Principles Emphasized by the Infant Doe Case." *Texas Tech Law Review* 14 (1983): 569–91.

Following an examination of the Bloomington, Indiana, Baby Doe case, the author concludes that cases of de facto infanticide occur, in part, through the application of family law principles. Principles of criminal law or constitutional rights, if considered, would protect the infant's rights and ensure aggressive treatment.

Brant, Jonathan, and Ann McNulty. "Treating Defective Newborns: The Ethical Dilemma." *Human Rights* 10 (Fall 1982): 35–37, 45–47.

The authors review a Massachusetts case in which a hospital went to court to secure a newborn's right to treatment against the parent's wishes. They conclude that the court's use of substituted judgment and the infant's best interest was no more than a weighing of the probability of the success of the treatment against its risks. They argue that other factors should also be considered in these cases.

Cosby, Michael G. "The Legacy of Infant Doe." *Baylor Law Review* 34 (Fall 1982): 699–715.

The author details the Bloomington, Indiana, case and then discusses the related legal problems of defining persons, establishing when life begins, and deciding whether quality-of-life factors should play a role in treatment decisions.

Curran, William. "Quality of Life and Treatment Decisions: The Canadian Law Reform Report." *New England Journal of Medicine* 310 (February 2, 1984): 297–98.

This article reviews the conclusions of the Canadian Law Reform Report concerning euthanasia, the right to refuse treatment, and obtaining consent to terminate treatment. It focuses especially on the role of physicians in making these decisions.

Cushing, Maureen. "Whose Best Interest? Parents vs. Child Rights." *American Journal of Nursing* 82 (February 1982): 313–14.

A nurse/lawyer reviews recent court cases which have involved questions of treatment for children. She also explains the tests courts use to determine the interests of children.

Department of Health and Human Services. "Procedures and Guidelines Relating to Health Care for Handicapped Infants." 45 Code of Federal Regulations, Part 84 (1984).

The final rules designed to enforce Section 504 of the Rehabilitation Act of 1973 with regard to nondiscrimination in the treatment of handicapped infants as published by HHS.

"Doctors May Have Authority to Withhold Life-Saving Measures." *Syracuse Herald-Journal*, September 17, 1984, A-12.

The New York State Health Commissioner proposes new legislation that would allow doctors and hospitals to withhold emergency treatment and heroic measures that would only prolong the suffering of terminal patients.

Fost, Norman. "Putting Hospitals on Notice." *Hastings Center Report* 12 (August 1982): 5–8.

Fost details the questions that arise concerning treatment of handicapped newborns and examines the role played by the U.S. Department of Health and Human Services in ensuring that infants are not denied treatment merely as a result of having a handicap.

Gray, Christopher B. "The Notion of Person for Medical Law." *Revue de Droit* 11 (1981): 341–415.

The author discusses the problem of when a person begins to exist and when one dies. He notes the stipulative, essential, and operational definitions in law and also addresses norms used in various Western countries. He concludes that an adequate standard must take account of continuing identity from conception on, but this identity can be compromised by extraordinary dependence on nonhuman support.

Gutheil, Thomas G., and Paul S. Appelbaum. "Substituted Judgment: Best Interests in Disguise." *Hastings Center Report* 13 (June 1983): 8-11.

The development of the doctrines of substituted judgment and best interests is examined with particular emphasis place on decisions made with the help of these legal standards.

Hentoff, Nat. "Troublemaking Babies and Pious Liberals." *Village Voice*, January 3, 1984, 8.

Hentoff discusses the problem of an uncertain future for handicapped infants, civil rights, and liberal journalists' responses to these matters.

Holder, Angela R. "Parents, Courts, and Refusal of Treatment." *Journal of Pediatrics* 103/4 (October 1983): 515–21.

Holder reviews a variety of judicial opinions to determine which factors seem important to judges who must decide whether parents will be allowed to make treatment decisions for their children. An analysis and history of the relevant regulations of the U.S. Department of Health and Human Services is also provided.

Horan, Dennis J., and Marianne E. Guerrini. "The Order to Treat: Judicial

Intervention in Benign Neglect of Defective Infants." *Linacre Quarterly* 49 (February 1982): 42–47.

The authors discuss decisions to refuse to treat infants who have some potential for survival. They also examine physicians' legal responsibility in those cases in which parents wish to withhold treatment.

In Re Claire C. Conroy, 98 N.J. 321, 486 A.2d. 1209 (1985).

In this far-reaching case on the rights of incompetent, terminally ill patients, the New Jersey Supreme Court detailed procedures which, when followed, will enable physicians to withhold treatment or end treatment for certain patients. The court refused to follow distinctions between providing normal life support and heroic treatment and between nontreatment and terminating active treatment. The court also decided that physicians could withdraw a feeding tube from a patient without incurring legal liability.

In the Matter of John Storar, In the *Matter of Philip Eichner*, 438 N.Y.S. 2d 362, 420 N.E.2d 64, *cert. den.* 454 v.s. 858 (1981).

In these combined cases the New York Court of Appeals ruled (1) that the guardian of Brother Fox could terminate medical support systems for Brother Fox on the basis of his previously expressed wishes and his permanent vegetative state, but that (2) the guardian of a terminally ill retarded man could not discontinue blood transfusions when the transfusions restored the patient to his normal state of alertness and did not cause him excessive pain.

Jarratt, David C. "Wrongful Life Recognized in Washington: *Harbeson v. Parke-Davis*." *Montana Law Review* 44 (Summer 1983): 291–96.

This article reviews a decision by the Washington Supreme Court which allows an infant with a birth defect to sue a drug company alleged to be responsible for causing the defect. Other cases in which this theory has been rejected are also discussed.

Kluge, Eike-Henner W. "The Euthanasia of Radically Defective Neonates: Some Statutory Considerations." *Dalhousie Law Journal* 6 (November 1980): 229–57.

Kluge argues that law and ethics should distinguish between "human beings" and "persons" so that hopelessly suffering infants may avoid the prolongation of their lives.

Levine, Carol, Anthony Gallo, and Bonnie Steinbock. "The Case of Baby Jane Doe." *Hastings Center Report* 14 (February 1984): 10–19.

This series of articles presents the history of the Long Island Baby Jane Doe case, an analysis of treatments and prognosis for infants suffering spina bifida, and a history of similar cases as they were resolved in the courts.

Magnet, Joseph Eliot. "Neonatal Intensive Care: The Dilemma for Medical Law." *Ottawa Law Review* 13 (1981): 345–55.

A Canadian law professor looks at decision making in twenty-nine intensive care centers. He finds that doctors rely not only on their medical expertise but also on personal data gathered by social workers. Canadian law is generally tolerant of the decisions then made by the physicians and families.

Margolick, David. "State High Court Says Death Occurs When Brain Halts." *New York Times,* October 31, 1984, p. A1.

This article reports on two cases decided by New York's Court of Appeals in which the court ruled that a person is legally dead when the brain ceases to function even though heart beat and respiration may be maintained by artificial methods.

McAllen, Peter F., and Richard Delgado. "Moral Experts in the Courtroom." *Hastings Center Report* 14 (February 1984): 27–34.

An examination of the role and ability of moral experts in presenting authoritative testimony in trials. The authors distinguish between normative ethics and descriptive ethics and suggest the latter is more appropriate for a courtroom witness.

McKinlay, John B., ed. *Law and Ethics in Health Care.* Cambridge, Mass.: MIT Press, 1982.

A collection of essays on the government's role in health care decisions, the ethical questions raised by new medical technologies, issues which arise in the treatment of critically ill patients, and the traditional role of law in medical practice.

Merkin, Leon. "Problem of 'Dying with Dignity.'" *New York State Journal of Medicine* 70 (January 1979): 101–6.

Merken examines "death with dignity" laws and medical cases of "terminal" patients who have survived. He then applies both in a discussion of euthanasia.

Portela, Carmen. "The *Elin Daniels* Case: An Examination of the Legal, Medical, and Ethical Considerations Posed When Parents and Doctors Disagree on Whether to Treat a Defective Newborn." *Forum* 18 (Summer 1983): 709–27.

In this Florida case the hospital won the right to treat an infant suffering from spina bifida. Portela reviews the case and argues that spina bifida patients should always be treated.

Richards, David A. J. "Constitutional Privacy, the Right to Die and the Meaning of Life: A Moral Analysis." *William and Mary Law Review* 22 (Spring 1981): 327–419.

Richards argues for a right to die, which be believes can be a logical extension of privacy rights now found in constitutional interpretations. He suggests that if legislatures cannot resolve these issues, then courts should develop defenses which would protect doctors from criminal liability in cases of passive euthanasia.

Robertson, John A. "Legal Norms and Procedures for Withholding Care from Incompetent Patients: The Role of Law in Passive Euthanasia." In *Frontiers in Medical Ethics: Applications in a Medical Setting*, ed. Virginia Abernethy, 99–113. Cambridge, Mass.: Ballinger Publishing Co., 1980.

The author argues that families, doctors and hospital review committees alone are not sufficient to protect the rights of incompetent persons. He suggests that due process requires that courts play a role in these decisions and discusses procedures and standards that courts might use.

———. "Involuntary Euthanasia of Defective Newborns: A Legal Analysis." *Stanford Law Review* 27 (January 1985): 213–69.

Following an analysis of criminal liability for those who participate in decisions to withhold treatment, Robertson concludes that parents, physicians and hospitals are often in violation of current laws. He argues that liability will be avoidable only when society can define a class of persons from whom care may be withheld and establish procedures for using such a definition.

Sargent, Kimball J. P. "Withholding Treatment from Defective Newborns: Substituted Judgment, Informed Consent, and the *Quinlan* Decision." *Gonzaga Law Review* 13 (1978): 781–811.

This article analyzes the rights of competent and incompetent adults to make treatment decisions and then discusses the applicability of these rights to newborn infants.

Severns v. Wilmington Medical Center, Inc., 421 A2d 1334 (Del. 1980), 425 A.2d 156 (Del. 1980).

The Delaware Supreme Court ruling that an uncompetent person may exercise substituted judgment through a legally appointed guardian and may, through the guardian, discontinue the use of life support technology.

Singer, Peter, and Helga Huhse. "The Future of Baby Doe." *New York Review of Books* 31 (March 1, 1984): 17–22.

The authors review *The Long Dying of Baby Andrew* by Robert and Peggy Stinson and examine the possible effects of intervention by the federal government into similar cases through the efforts of the Department of Health and Human Services.

Spicker, Stuart F., and others, eds. *The Law-Medicine Relation: A Philosophical Exploration.* Boston: D. Reidel Publishing Co., 1981.

Papers from a symposium on the topic cited. Of particular interest are discussions of legal rights in health care, criteria and procedures for withholding ethical and legal responsibility given uncertainty in prognosis, and wrongful life cases.

Suber, Daniel G., and William J. Tabor. "Withholding of Life-Sustaining Treatment from the Terminally Ill, Incompetent Patient: Who Decides?" *Journal of the American Medical Association* 248 (November 19, 1982): 2431–32.

    The authors review recent court cases, the need for judicial approval and the risk of liability to physicians faced with treatment decisions for incompetent patients.

Taub, Sheila. "Withholding Treatment from Defective Newborns." *Law, Medicine and Health Care* 10 (February 1982): 4–10.

    Recent court cases involving the treatment of infants born with birth defects are reviewed. Taub also discusses the legal distinction between withholding and terminating treatment and the responsibility of the parties for decisions in this kind of case.

Weber v. Stony Brook Hospital, et al. 95 A.D.2d 587 (1983)

    The trial court in this, the Baby Jane Doe Case, appointed a guardian ad litem for the child and directed that surgery be performed. On appeal, the Appellate Division reversed the trial court's decision in its entirety and ruled that the parents had made reasonable and informed decisions concerning the best treatment for their daughter.

Weber v. Stony Brook Hospital et al. 60 N.Y.2d 208 (1983)

    New York's highest court, the Court of Appeals, affirmed the decision of the Appellate Division and dismissed the Baby Jane Doe case.

3. Economic Considerations: Allocation of Resources

Research on cost considerations is not as robust or helpful as the literatures in law and moral philosophy. Even the yearly aggregate expenditure on neonatal nurseries in the United States is an estimate, not a precise figure. Also, the use of normative theory to justify limiting medical expenditures is tentative, by no means conclusive and often not even persuasive. The references listed here are the ones I found most useful in trying to think clearly about medical costs in neonatology. The Blue Cross study I use in chapter 5 is described in the Kaufman and Shepard piece.

Bloom, Bernard S. "Changing Infant Mortality: The Need to Spend More While Getting Less." *Pediatrics* 73 (June 1984): 862–66.

    Infant mortality is characterized by diminishing marginal returns. Bloom raises questions of where to draw lines when allocating ever more costly treatments to infant patients.

Freedman, Benjamin. "The Eyes of the Beholders: Roles and the Distribution of Scarce Medical Resources." *Theoretical Medicine* 4 (Fall 1982): 92–111.

> Freedman examines resource allocations as they would be made by different participants in health care decisions, from practitioners to policymakers. He suggests that it is possible to pool these differing perspectives and arrive at a just allocation of medical resources.

Hewetson, Debra S. "Scarce Medical Resource Allocation—The Case of First Impression: A Hypothetical Opinion of the Twelfth Circuit United States Courts of Appeals." *Journal of Legal Medicine* 3 (June 1982): 295–315.

> Hewetson creates a situation in which a hospital uses a review board to allocate scarce resources and finds itself facing a suit from a patient's estate in which the patient claims a violation of due process under the Constitution.

Hoppe, Ruth B. "Decision Theory and Health Resource Allocations." *Theoretical Medicine* 4 (June 1983): 193–206.

> The ethical implications of applying cost utility analysis to decisions regarding the distribution of medical resources.

Kaufman, Susan L., and Donald S. Shepard. "Costs of Neonatal Intensive Care by Day of Stay." *Inquiry* 19 (Summer 1982): 167–78.

> A study of the costs of care for low birth-weight infants broken down by component costs, per day costs, and costs per length of stay.

Kilner, John F. "A Moral Allocation of Scarce Medical Resources." *Journal of Religious Ethics* 9 (Fall 1981): 245–85.

> Kilner defines a just policy for the allocation of medical resources based on both a right to life and considerations of equality and need. He then examines possible exceptions to his theory of justice and explains why they should be rejected or accepted, e.g., life expectancy or social merit.

———. "Who Shall Be Saved? An African Answer." *Hastings Center Report* 14 (June 1984): 18–21.

> Kilner presents the results of his research into the microallocation of medical resources in Kenya. Persons of differing cultures have widely different views on how to value lives when insufficient resources are available for all.

McCarthy, John T., and others. "Who Pays the Bill for Neonatal Intensive Care?" *Journal of Pediatrics* 95 (1979): 755–62.

> This study details neonatal care costs and the share of those costs paid by parents, hospitals and insurers.

McIntyre, Keven M., Robert C. Benfari, and Margaret Pabst Battin. "Two

Cardiac Arrests, One Medical Team." *Hastings Center Report* 12 (April 1982): 24–25.

The authors use a hypothetical case to discuss the allocation of treatment and medical resources. The "first come, first served" standard is compared with other standards that involve likelihood of success and the social costs involved in treatment.

Menzel, Paul T. *A Philosophy of Health Care Economics in America.* New Haven, Conn.: Yale University Press, 1983.

The author introduces a philosophical framework within which he develops an ideal-type model of "costworthy" health care. The model is used to examine a number of issues in health care costs.

Pomerance, Jeffrey J., and others. "Cost of Living for Infants Weighing 1000 Grams or Less at Birth." *Pediatrics* 61 (June 1978): 908–10.

This study provides average and total hospital cost data for low birth-weight infants. The cases are segregated by those who died, those who survived, and those survivors who can be termed "normal."

Strong, Carson. "The Tiniest Newborns." *Hastings Center Report* 13 (February 1983): 14–19.

Strong examines treatment, treatment costs, and survival rates for low birth-weight infants. He also reviews arguments for avoiding aggressive treatment for these infants and finds them unconvincing. He asserts that current practices are justifiable.

Walker, Donna-Jean B., and others. "Cost-Benefit Analysis of Neonatal Intensive Care for Infants Weighing Less Than 1000 Grams at Birth." *Pediatrics* 74 (July 1984): 20–25.

Hospital costs for low birth-weight infants demonstrate an inverse correlation between weight and cost. The authors compare costs per weight (by class) and the expected lifetime income of the survivors and conclude that intensive care may not be justified for neonates weighing less than 900 grams at birth.

4. Ethics, Philosophy, and Moral Decision Making

The philosophical literature in biomedical ethics is exciting and vast. The almost exponential growth rate of excellent contributions represents a turn to issues since the mid-1970s. Philosophers are now inclined to apply normative theory to social problems and practices, and not simply analyze moral discourse. The results are so interesting that one wonders why philosophy dwelled so long on the meanings of moral terms. I have included here a number of fine anthologies, including Tom Beauchamp's various collections. Also note the articles on rights, the most interesting of which are those by Charvet and Louden. See also the arguments of Oldenquist on moral communities. My reliance on "harm" owes much to John Stuart Mill's *On Liberty*. But also see the quite different interpretations of "harm" by Harman and Jonsen ("Do No Harm").

Abernethy, Virginia, ed. *Frontiers in Medical Ethics*. Cambridge, Mass.: Ballinger Publishing Co., 1980.

These essays by a number of noted authors in medical ethics present the principal problems that confront doctors, patients, and those who would speak for patients. The essays also examine the ethicist's role in providing counsel to those facing decisions in health settings.

Abrams, Natalie, and Michael D. Buckner, eds. *Medical Ethics: A Clinical Textbook and Reference for the Health Care Professions*. Cambridge, Mass.: MIT Press, 1983.

A collection of the standard articles on clinical ethics to which are added seventy-four clinical case studies, ten contemporary professional codes of ethics, six classic legal cases, and two indexes.

Agich, George, ed. *Responsibility in Health Care*. Dordrecht, Holland: D. Reidel Publishing Co., 1982.

Writings on responsibility in the provision of health care in team settings. Topics include integrity, legal responsibility, medical authority, and doctor-patient relationships.

American Medical Association. *Current Opinions of the Judicial Council of the American Medical Association*. Chicago: American Medical Association, 1982.

This booklet contains the official opinion of the AMA on various issues in medical ethics. Of special interest is the view that parents should be presumed to have their children's best interests in mind when making treatment decisions. Doctors who have evidence to the contrary are expected to assert themselves strongly during consultation. The AMA also sees a role for quality-of-life factors in treatment decisions.

Arras, John D. "Toward an Ethic of Ambiguity." *Hastings Center Report* 14 (April 1984): 25–33.

The Reagan administration adopted a "nondiscrimination principle" to guide the medical community in its treatment of handicapped newborns. Arras searches for the practical substance of such a principle and finds that it does not fulfill the best interest of the children and is not consistent with other principles which could be used to make treatment decisions.

Basson, Mare, Rachel Lipson, and Doreen Ganos, eds. *Troubling Problems in Medical Ethics*. New York: Alan R. Liss, 1981.

The proceedings of the 1980 and 1981 University of Michigan

Conferences on Ethics, Humanism, and Medicine. The authors attempt to eliminate normative theory and focus instead on the moral imperatives of particular cases. Issues discussed include competency, confidentiality, consent, and nonresuscitation.

Battin, Margaret P. "Non-Patient Decision Making in Medicine: The Eclipse of Altruism." *Journal of Medicine and Philosophy* 10, no. 1 (February 1985): 19–44.

Battin argues that transferring decision making from the patient to professional or lay decision makers who are assessing the interests of the patient tends to preclude altruistic choices on the part of the patient. Thus decisions that should properly be made by the patient, such as refusing life-prolonging treatment, are instead made by others who may not make a decision preferred by the patient.

Beauchamp, Tom L. "A Reply to Rachels on Active and Passive Euthanasia." In Tom L. Beauchamp and Terry Pinkard, eds., *Ethics and Public Policy*, (Englewood Cliffs, N.J.: Prentice-Hall, 1983), 318–30.

The author distinguishes between passive and active euthanasia, and then argues that endorsing euthanasia will begin a slide toward other forms of justified killing and erode principles that protect human life.

Beauchamp, Tom L., and James F. Childress. *Principles of Biomedical Ethics.* 2d Edition. New York: Oxford University Press, 1983.

Beauchamp and Childress define ethical principles which they argue should apply broadly to all types of moral and biomedical problems. In doing so they discuss utilitarianism and deontological theories, principles of autonomy, nonmaleficence, beneficence, and justice as they apply to medical ethics.

Beauchamp, Tom, and Walter LeRoy, eds. *Contemporary Issues in Bioethics.* Belmont, Cal.: Wadsworth Publishing Co., 1982.

The authors (Beauchamp especially) articulate an applied ethics model that attempts to assign principles of general normative theory to medical circumstances, accommodating in the assignment certain conceptual idiosyncrasies of the institutions of medicine.

Beauchamp, Tom L., and Seymour Perin, eds. *Ethical Issues in Death and Dying.* Englewood Cliffs, N.J.: Prentice-Hall, 1978.

A vast collection of articles by noted authors on the definition of death, the rights of dying patients, euthanasia, and the justification of suicide.

Bell, Nora K. "Triage in Medical Practices: An Unacceptable Model?" *Social Science and Medicine* 15 (1981): 151–56.

Triage, which the author sees as perhaps a useful principle in wartime, cannot be successfully used in normal medical circumstances. Bell argues that triage is inconsistent with accepted ideas concerning the value of life in medical settings.

————, ed. *Who Decides?* Clifton: Humana Press, 1982.
Essays on personal autonomy, refusing treatment and withdrawing treatment, the use of "heroic" methods, and an introduction on rights in medical settings.

Bell, N. K., and Loewer, B. M "What is Wrong with 'Wrongful Life' Cases?" *Journal of Medicine and Philosophy*, 10, no. 2 (May 1985): 127–45.
The authors attempt to rebut arguments often used to disallow "wrongful life" cases, such as the senselessness of claiming that one would be better off if one had never existed or the impossibility of assessing the extent to which one has been damaged by being brought into existence, and suggest a procedure for determining damages in "wrongful life" cases.

Bolsen, Barbara. "Theraputic Choices Not Always Predictable." *Journal of the American Medical Association* 247 (March 5, 1982): 1231–35.
Bolsen reports on three studies of medical practices. Of interest here is the conclusion that decisions by patients were strongly influenced by the way choices were presented—whether in terms of probability of death or probability of survival. In cancer cases choices were also influenced by specification or nonspecification of the method of treatment.

Bondeson, William, and others, eds. *New Knowledge in the Biomedical Sciences: Some Moral Implications of Its Acquisition, Possession, and Use.* Boston: D. Reidel Publishing Co., 1982.
This volume contains essays relating the development of technology to moral issues in health care. Topics include the costs of knowledge, the social control of technology, the distribution of technology via different economic models, and the physician's role as a moral force in decision making.

Boorse, Christopher. "Health as a Theoretical Concept." *Philosophy of Science* 44 (December 1977): 542–73.
"Health" is best viewed as a value-free theoretical concept, according to Boorse. He argues that those who see health as value-laden are mistaken. Instead he suggests that the concept be understood in terms of statistically normal physiological functioning. Disease and injury reduce functional abilities below normal levels; health care restores abilities to normal levels.

Brandt, Richard, "Defective Newborns and the Morality of Termination." In Marvin Kohl, ed., *Infanticide and the Value of Life* (Buffalo, N.Y.: Prometheus Books, 1978), 46–60.

The author argues that involuntary euthanasia, either active or passive, is warranted for seriously defective newborns. Those decisions to terminate life should be made within ten days after the birth of an infant.

Buchanan, Allen. "Medical Paternalism." *Philosophy and Public Affairs* 7 (Summer 1978): 370–90.

Physicians, according to Buchanan, use paternalistic arguments to dominate decision making on medical treatment. Buchanan argues that medical paternalism is not warranted and that one need not rely on a theory of the moral rights of patients to show that it is not.

Cassel, Eric J. "The Nature of Suffering and the Goals of Medicine." *New England Journal of Medicine* 306 (March 18, 1982): 639–45.

Cassel describes the nature and causes of suffering and distinguishes between suffering and physical distress. He then questions some uses of medical techniques and argues that one purpose of medicine is to relieve suffering. Medicine fails when it results in increased or prolonged suffering.

Charvet, John. "A Critique of Human Rights." In *Nomos XXIII: Human Rights*, ed. Roland Pennock and John W. Chapman, 31–51. New York: New York University Press, 1981.

The Charvet summary argues that the essential idea of human rights—a grounding of men's claims on man's own nature—is incoherent. The incoherence issues from a failure to recognize differences between a moral self and a particular self in each individual. The two selves can be reconciled only in a communal structure creating more general rights and duties for its members.

Childress, James F. *Priorities in Biomedical Ethics*. Philadelphia: Westminister Press, 1981.

Childress develops arguments on a variety of topics, including the just use of paternalism, decisions to allow people to die, and the allocation of medical resources. His goal is to determine how principles such as respecting others and not harming them can be used in decision making when they appear to offer conflicting guidance.

———. "Triage in Neonatal Intensive Care: The Limitations of a Metaphor." *Virginia Law Review* 69 (April 1983): 547–61.

Childress argues against triage and suggests instead the use of randomization or queuing in the allocation of medical resources. He also discusses quality of life factors, the distinction between withholding and withdrawing treatment, and medical utility as opposed to social utility.

Coburn, Robert D. "Morality and the Defective Newborn." *Journal of Medicine and Philosophy* 5 (December 1980): 340–57.

Coburn attempts to demonstrate that principles regarding the moral treatment of defective newborns can be articulated with a reliance on rights based on utilitarian theories. He argues for two principles which would deny the termination of life and two which would allow it on the basis of the potential for life, the expected quality of life, and the anticipated effect of that life on others.

Cohen, Cynthia B. "'Quality of Life' and the Analogy with the Nazis." *Journal of Medicine and Philosophy* 8 (May 1983): 113–36.

Cohen argues that "quality of life" has been misconstrued by its opponents. The term does not properly refer to the value of life but to the well-being of individuals. Quality-of-life considerations should therefore form a part of treatment decisions.

Diamond, Eugene F. "The AMA and Infanticide: An Unfortunate Guideline." *Linacre Quarterly* 48 (August 1981): 207–11.

Diamond offers criticism of an opinion of the Judicial Council of the AMA which suggests that doctors defer to the wishes of parents when treating birth-defective infants. This opinion, in Diamond's view, ignores the moral and legal responsibilities of physicians.

Duff, Raymond S., and A. G. M. Campbell. "Moral and Ethical Dilemmas in the Special-Care Nursery." *New England Journal of Medicine* 289 (October 25, 1973): 890–94.

An investigation of nearly 300 deaths in a special care nursery revealed that 14 percent were related to decisions to withhold treatment. Duff and Campbell examine these decisions and the basis of moral decision making among physicians and families.

Dworkin, Gerald. "Paternalism." *The Monist* 56 (January 1972): 64–84.

Dworkin argues that paternalism, the interference with an individual's liberty for the individual's own welfare or the welfare of society, can be justified under certain circumstances. He suggests that laws which are paternalistic can be seen as insurance against potentially dangerous and irreversible acts, and argues that rational people will find paternalistic laws—seen in this light—justified when both the potential harm and the probability of harm is great.

Fleischman, Alan R., and Thomas H. Murray. "Ethics Committees for Infants Doe?" *Hastings Center Report* 13 (December 1983): 5–9.

Ethics committees could provide valuable guidance on treatment decisions, according to the authors, who detail the possible roles for these committees in hospitals.

Harman, John D. "Harm, Consent and Distress." *Journal of Value Inquiry* 15 (1981): 293–309.

The author discusses some difficulties in the relations between harm and consent. He proposes a distress definition of harm to overcome these difficulties. He also argues that harm-as-distress modifies arguments over the legitimacy of paternalistic legislation.

————. "Rights and Social Freedom." *Metaphilosophy* 14 (July–October 1983), 209–24.

A discussion of the difficulties that follow from assuming that rights are both moral and legal *and* that rights can apply to social freedom issues.

Humber, James M., and Robert F. Almeder, eds. *Biomedical Ethics and the Law.* 2d ed. New York: Plenum Press, 1979.

The last section of this volume contains articles that address some of the questions concerning ethics, dying, active and passive euthanasia, the use of heroic measures, and the allocation of life-saving technology.

Infant Bioethics Task Force and Consultants. "Guidelines for Bioethics Committees." *Pediatrics* 74 (August 1984): 306–10.

The American Academy of Pediatrics recommends that hospitals establish Infant Bioethics Committees to provide advice on treatment decisions. The function, structure, and membership of such committees is described in these guidelines.

Johnson, Paul R. "Selective Nontreatment and Spina Bifida: A Case Study in Ethical Theory and Application." *Bioethics Quarterly* 3 (Summer 1982): 91–111.

Johnson uses quality-of-life standards in his argument on when nontreatment of newborns is morally justified. He claims that when the potential for relationships with others is absent, a negative quality of life exists and is an adequate reason for withholding treatment.

Jonsen, Albert R. "Do No Harm." *Annals of Internal Medicine* 88 (1978): 827.

A helpful discussion of various senses of harm—e.g., harm versus wrongful harm—in medical therapy.

Jonsen, Albert R., Mark Siegler, and William J. Windslade. *Clinical Ethics: A Practical Approach to Ethical Decisions in Clinical Medicine.* New York: Macmillan Publishing Co., 1982.

The authors see clinical medicine as governed by three internal models: (1) acute, where the goal is the cure and rehabilitation of patients with acute life-threatening diseases; (2) care, where the goal is palliative treatment for those with chronic lethal diseases; and (3) cope, where the goal is enabling patients with chronic debilitating diseases to live the most meaningful and autonomous existence compatible with their condition.

Kaminski, Mitchell V., Jr. "Humanism in Hyperalimentation." *Journal of Perenteral and Enteral Nutrition* 5 (1981): 1–6.

The author examines the role of humanitarian principles in decisions regarding the provision of nutrition to seriously ill patients. He discusses when to begin and when to discontinue treatment and the role of the patient and family in making these decisions.

Kass, Leon R. "Regarding the End of Medicine and the Pursuit of Health." *The Public Interest*, no. 40 (Summer 1975): 11–42.

The author argues that health is the proper end of medicine, not the prolongation of life or the prevention of death. He defines health in terms of the Greek notions of *function* and *wholeness*, i.e., a well-working of the whole organism.

Katz, Jay. "Why Doctors Don't Disclose Uncertainty." *Hastings Center Report* 14 (February 1984): 35–44.

Katz discusses the social and psychological reasons for doctors' failure to admit the fallibility and uncertainty in their practice.

Leenen, H. J. J. "Selection of Patients." *Journal of Medical Ethics* 8 (March 1982): 33–36.

Leenen reviews possible systems for use in the selection of patients for life-sustaining resources. He also establishes criteria and examines values that might be used as the basis for such decisions.

Levine, Carol. "Questions and (Some Very Tentative) Answers about Hospital Ethics Committees." *Hastings Center Report* 14 (June 1984): 9–11.

Levine defines and gives data on hospital ethics committees. She also discusses the role and benefits that these committees may bring to treatment decisions.

Longino, Preston H., Jr. "Withholding Treatment from Defective Newborns: Who Decides and on What Criteria?" *University of Kansas Law Review* 31 (Spring 1983): 377–407.

Longino first attempts to identify when treatment might reasonably be withheld from newborns. He uses standards such as the infant's best interest, the quality of life, and medical feasibility. He then tries to identify the proper role of parents, physicians, ethics committees, and courts in applying these standards.

Loudon, Robert B. "Rights Infatuation and the Impoverishment of Moral Theory." *Journal of Value Inquiry* 17 (1983): 17–87.

A survey of rights theories and a recognition that the linking of rights with autonomy, choice, dignity, reflects a basic truth about morality. However, the author is critical about the capacities of rights to make distinctions among permitted actions. This conceptual impoverishment leads to bizarre conclusions when rights are used in situations requiring virtues, ends, and duties.

Lynn, Joanne, and James F. Childress. "Must Patients Always Be Given Food and Water?" *Hastings Center Report* 13 (October 1983): 17–21.

> According to the authors, there should be a presumption in favor of giving patients nutrition and fluids. There are, however, a limited number of cases in which it is not in the best interest of the patient to receive nourishment. They specifically discuss the Infant Doe case and the case of Claire Conroy later decided by the New Jersey Supreme Court.

Lyon, Jeff. *Playing God in the Nursery.* New York: Norton, 1985.

> A journalist reports on the political and moral issues in neonatology. In an artful blend of facts and theories, Lyon defends the current reliance on parents and doctors for therapy decisions against the use of the legal system.

MacMillan, Elizabeth S. "Birth Defective Infants: A Standard for Nontreatment Decisions." *Standford Law Review* 30 (February 1978): 599–633.

> Infants, parents, and the state all have conflicting interests in treatment decisions. The author examines various standards that might be used by these parties, rejects the use of quality-of-life considerations, and suggests medical feasibility as an alternative.

McCarthy, Rev. Donald G. "Treating Defective Newborns: Who Judges Extraordinary Means?" *Hospital Progress* 62 (December 1981): 45–49, 54.

> McCarthy argues that parents are primarily responsible for treatment decisions of newborns because they have the emotional ties which are important when deciding for another. Doctors, however, can best determine when heroic treatment methods are likely to offer long-term health to the infant. They have moral obligations, therefore, to guide parents' decisions and overrule them when necessary to preserve the life of the infant.

McConnell, Terrence. "Treatment without Consent." In *The Life Sciences and Human Values,* ed. James B. Wilbur. Proceedings of the 13th Conference on Value Inquiry, State University of New York at Geneseo, 1979.

> A discussion of cases in which medical treatment without consent is justified, and an exploration via Dworkin and Mill of actual versus intended desires with some of the problems that attach to the use of intended desires.

McNeil, Barbara J., and others. "On the Elicitation of Preferences for Alternative Therapies." *New England Journal of Medicine* 306 (May 27, 1982): 1259–62.

> The results of a study of decision making by surrogate patients. Decisions were greatly influenced by preexisting ideas, by the use of

statistics in informing the "patients," by whether the treatments were identified, and by whether the outcomes were described in terms of death or survival.

Moskop, John C. "Rawlsian Justice and a Human Right to Health Care." *Journal of Medicine and Philosophy* 8 (November 1983): 329–38.
    Moskop examines Rawls's theory of justice and suggests that health care should not be considered a human right but rather a social ideal which may then lead to the development of specific legal rights.

Murray, Thomas H. "The Final Anticlimatic Rule on Baby Doe." *The Hastings Center Report* 15 (June 1985): 5–10.
    Murray argues that the final set of federal regulations on the care of disabled infants is vague and reflects the ambivalence of American society toward both the law and protection of such infants.

Nursing Life Magazine. "The Right to Die, Part 2: On Deciding Whether to Treat Seriously Ill Newborns." *Nursing Life*, (March–April 1984, 45–52.
    A summary of a poll of over 3500 nurses regarding the practice of allowing seriously ill or deformed infants to die. The poll indicates that nurses generally favor this practice, but their comments indicate a reluctance to form general rules for all cases. Participants also expressed uncertainty on when a deformed child could be expected to live a meaningful life.

Oldenquist, Andrew. "Loyalties." *Journal of Philosophy*, April 1982, 173–93.
    The author develops a case for group loyalty as essential to a moral community. He argues that we universalize moral judgments, treat equals equally, protect the common good, and in general employ impersonal morality only within moral domains established by a kind of tribal loyalty.

Onondaga County Medical Society. "Guidelines for 'Do Not Resuscitate.'" *Bulletin of the Onondaga County Medical Society* 46 (October 1982): 11.
    These guidelines detail procedures for physicians who wish to write and implement a 'do not resuscitate' order for a patient.

President's Commission for the Study of Ethical Problems in Medicine and Biomedical and Behavioral Research. *Deciding to Forego Life-Sustaining Treatment.* Washington: U.S. Government Printing Office, 1983.
    The commission concludes that patients can give informed consent to the termination of life-supporting treatment. An incompetent patient's interests can be accommodated when those making therapy decisions use existing legal procedures for determining the patient's best interest.

The President's Commission for the Study of Ethical Problems in Medicine and Biomedical and Behavioral Research. *Making Health Care Decisions*. 3 vols. Washington: U.S. Government Printing Office, 1982.

This report addresses the ability of patients and doctors to make health care decisions based on the informed consent of autonomous parties. The report specifically discusses cultural problems, the issues raised by incompetent patients and minors, and includes the results of empirical studies on physician-patient communication.

Purtillo, Ruth, and Christine Gassel. *Ethical Dimensions in the Health Professions*. Philadephia: W. B. Saunders Co., 1981.

The authors develop a pragmatic, case-oriented approach to medical ethics that stresses a four-step procedure: (1) gather as much information as possible; (2) determine the nature of the ethical dilemma; (3) decide what should be done and how best to do it; and (4) do it.

Quinlan, Joseph, and Julia Quinlan, with Phyllis Battele. *Karen Ann: The Quinlans Tell Their Story*. New York: Doubleday, 1977.

The parents of Karen Ann Quinlan relate their views on their daughter's condition and the therapy decisions they made.

Rachels, James. "Active and Passive Euthanasia." *New England Journal of Medicine* 292 (January 1975): 78–80.

The author maintains that it is better to kill a baby painlessly than to allow a slow and painful death through dehydration and infection. Further, the quality of a baby's life should be a deciding factor in treatment decisions.

Randal, Judith. "Are Ethics Committees Alive and Well?" *Hastings Center Report* 13 (December 1983): 10–12.

A short history of the role of ethics committees is presented along with a survey of their use in hospitals. Randal concludes that much confusion still surrounds these bodies and the place they have in treatment decisions.

Rolston, Holmes. "The Irreversibly Comatose: Respect for the Subhuman in Human Life." *Journal of Medicine and Philosophy* 7 (November 1982):337–54.

Is there a duty to preserve life in the absence of personal consciousness? Rolston argues that in some cases there is and then uses his argument to address questions of active versus passive euthanasia and ordinary versus extraordinary treatment of comatose patients.

Ross, Val. "The 'Right to Die' Debate." *World Press Review* 31 (February 1984): 32–33.

Ross explains some of the issues surrounding the technical ability to keep terminal patients alive and the practice of euthanasia in Canadian Hospitals.

Rudolph, Claire S. "Regionalized Perinatal Services." *Maxwell News and Notes* 19 (1984): 2–3.

The author describes the development of perinatal care facilities which provide services to potentially high-risk pregnant women.

Scott, Charles E., and others. "Simulated Medical Ethics Rounds: Decision for a Newborn Infant." In *Frontiers in Medical Ethics: Applications in a Medical Setting*, ed. Virginia Abernathy, 121–37. Cambridge, Ma.: Ballinger Publishing Co., 1980.

Health practitioners discuss a hypothetical case in a special care nursery with philosophers, a chaplain, and a lawyer. The discussion is noteworthy for the doctors' belief that informed consent cannot be given by parents. The doctors see their role as guiding the parents to accept professional judgments.

Shaw, Anthony. "Defining the Quality of Life." *Hasting Center Report* 7 (October 1977): 11.

Shaw attempts to formalize the elements which constitute what we mean by the "quality of life" and argues that these elements are often not considered by medical practitioners.

Shaw, Anthony, Judson G. Randolph, and Babara Manard. "Ethical Issues in Pediatric Surgery: A National Survey of Pediatricians and Pediatric Surgeons." *Pediatrics* 60 (October, 1977): 588–99.

This survey examines doctors' opinions regarding the initiation of treatment, the role of parents in making treatment decisions for childrens, and the withholding or termination of treatment. Specific questions explored are which diseases or combinations of diseases doctors think should go untreated, whether a physician should see a court order to initiate treatment for certain diseases over parents' objections, and whether courts or judges should play a role in "normal" treatment decisions.

Shelp, Earl E., ed. *Beneficence and Health Care*. Boston: D. Reidel Publishing Co., 1982.

This series of essays first seeks to define beneficence in accordance with a variety of ethical and religious traditions. The definitions are then taken into the health care discussion as the authors attempt to show how a patient can benefit from health care decisions in hard cases.

———. *Philosophy and Medicine: Beneficence and Health Care*, vol. 2 Boston: D. Reidel Publishing Co., 1982.

These essays examine the relationship between beneficense and normative questions in health care. Topics include the nature of the

moral duty of beneficence, its history in medicine, and its application in medical setting.

Singer, Peter. "All Animals Are Equal." *Philosophical Exchange* 2, no. 1
(1974).

The author maintains that any characteristic that covers all humans will be possessed by some animals. It follows that sentience is
a better principle of action than those principles that seem to demarcate humans as a separate species. The rights of animals are founded
in their capacity to suffer.

————. *Practical Ethics.* New York: Cambridge University Press, 1979.

Singer's book is a collection of thoughtful essays that include a
discussion of the value of human life and the problems of assigning
value to conscious life. He also discusses euthanasia, including
arguments for and against passive and active euthanasia.

Strong, Carson, "The Neonatologists' Duty to Patient and Parents." *Hastings Center Report* 14 (August 1984): 10–16.

Policymakers have recently declared that the interests of infants
should prevail when treatment decisions concerning them are
made. Strong discusses several reasons why, when doctors and
parents disagree, the physician's view of the child's best interests
may be important to decision making.

Swazey, Judith P. "To Treat or Not to Treat: The Search for Principled
Decisions." In *Frontiers in Medical Ethics: Applications in a Medical
Setting,* ed. Virginia Abernethy. Cambridge, Mass.: Ballinger Pub-
lishing Co., 1980.

Swazey claims that the discussion of treatment decisions in
medical ethics suffers from a lack of semantic and analytic clarity.
She explores generally the rights and responsibilities of parties
involved in making decisions to provide or withhold treatment.

Twycross, Robert G. "Debate: Euthanasia—A Physician's Viewpoint" (includes commentary by Nancy Lindmerer). *Journal of Medical Ethics* 8
(June 1982): 86–95.

Changes in medical education, not changes in legal standards,
are needed in order in ensure that terminally ill patients are cared for
with compassion and respect for life. Twycross argues that current
laws which ban euthanasia need no amendment.

Vinogradov, Sophia, Joe E. Thornton, A-J Rock Levinson, and Michael L.
Callen. "If I Have AIDS, Then Let Me Die Now!" *Hastings Center
Report* 14 (February 1984): 24–26.

Psychiatrists and several activists concerned with the rights of
terminally ill patients discuss the case history of an AIDS victim who
refused treatment.

254   Bibliography

Walton, Douglas N. "On Allowing Something to Happen." *Man and Medicine* 5 (1980): 167–88.

A philosopher enters the debate on active and passive euthanasia with an examination of the moral relevance of the distinction between causing an event and allowing an event to occur.

Wanzer, Sidney H., and others. "The Physician's Responsibility toward Hopelessly Ill Patients." *New England Journal of Medicine* 310 (April 12, 1984): 955–59.

A group of physicians attempts to establish guidelines for use by the medical community in terminating the use of life support technology.

Zembat, Jane S. "A Limited Defense of Medical Paternalism." In *The Life Science and Human Values*, ed. James B. Wilbur. Proceedings of the 13th Conference on Value Inquiry, State University of New York at Geneseo, 1979.

A discussion of paternalism which concludes that paternalism is justified "when autonomy is protected to a much greater degree than it would be if a nonpaternalistic position were accepted" (p. 156).

Zimrin, Joseph G. "Medical Judgment vs. Court Imposed Rules in the Treatment of Terminally Ill Patients." *New York State Journal of Medicine* 81 (May 1981): 951–54.

Zimring questions the standards enunciated in *In the Matter of Brother Joseph Fox* in light of the facts and ethical values that govern a physician's judgment in such a case.

5. Decision Theory and Personhood

The remarks on decision theory that open chapter 5 and on elaborate therapy decisions in chapter 11 refer to a literature that, in the main, agrees that Bayesian decision-rules are rational to employ in conditions of risk, perhaps in conditions of uncertainty, while maximin and maximax decision-rules do well in conditions of uncertainty, are less rational in conditions of risk or certainty. The literature also provides various elegant models of bounded rationality to replace the classical rationality found in modern equilibrium theory: a "satisficing" version of rationality developed on imperfect information, information costs, and a static environment, and game-theoretic rationalities in which decisions are made on strategic rather than parametric grounds (the environment is variable). More recent experiments have suggested a stronger role for heuristics in rational actions than anticipated. See the works listed below by Elster (for the description of a shift to game-theoretic rationalities), Simon (for "satisficing" rationality), and Tversky and Kahneman (for the experiments demonstrating the importance of heuristics in decisions). The use of Bayesian decision-rules is described in most introductory texts on decision theory and/or probability theory, for example R. M. Thrall, C. H. Coombes, and R. L. Davis, eds., *Decision Processes*(New York: John Wiley, 1954); R. Duncan Luce and Howard Raiffe, *Games and Decisions* (New York: John Wiley, 1957); and R. C. Jeffrey, *The Logic of Decision* (New York: McGraw-Hill, 1965). Also the paragraph on open concepts on page 212 is influenced by the Gallie article below.

Let me note briefly that the philosophical literature on personhood does not exist in any satisfactory form, through the two volumes by MacMurray represent some thoughtful exercises on this subject.

Elster, Jon. *Logic and Society*. New York: John Wiley, 1978.
> An imaginative survey and discussion of rational choice theory and a number of social theories and practices.

Fletcher, Joseph. "Indicators of Humanhood: A Tentative Profile of Man." *Hastings Center Report* 2 (November 1972): 1–4.
> An attempt to list essential characteristics of personhood and also to refute some candidates for that list.

———. "Four Indicators of Humanhood—The Enquiry Matures." *Hastings Center Report* December 4 (1974): 4–7.
> Continuing the enquiry begun in 1972, Fletcher refines essential human features to this list of four: neocortical function, self-consciousness, relational ability, and happiness.

Gallie, W. B. "Essentially Contested Concepts." *Proceedings of the Aristotelian Society*, 1955, 167–98.
> The early and classic statement on how concepts can be essentially contestable (or open to interpretation in legitimately competing ways).

Jones, James. *Bad Blood*. New York: The Free Press, 1981.
> A study of the medical study of syphilis victims that required not treating the control group of victims.

MacMurray, John. *The Self as Agent*. London: Faber & Faber, 1953.
> MacMurray criticizes the traditions of philosophy which focus on the individual as a reflective, isolated, knowing subject and instead suggests that the self be seen as an actor. Altered concepts of causality and knowledge result: theories of knowledge become subordinate to theories of action.

———. *Persons in Relation*. London: Faber & Faber, 1954.
> In this second volume, MacMurray elaborates on the concept of personhood that results from his view of the person as actor. Personal life is seen in terms of mutual relationships so that human life is characterized not simply by an "I" but by a "you and I."

Morris, Colin. *The Discovery of the Individual, 1050–1200*. New York: Harper & Row, 1972.
    Morris examines literary, artistic, and historical sources to find the origin of the concept of the individual in the history of thought.

Simon, Herbert. 1982. *Models of Bounded Rationality*. Cambridge, Mass.: MIT Press.

Tversky, Amos, and Daniel Kahneman. 1982. *Judgment Under Uncertainty: Heuristics and Biases*. Cambridge: Cambridge.

Index

Italicized page numbers refer to entries in the Glossary. Names of hospitals, patients and their families, hospital staff, and physicians (defined below as "baby," "nurse," "physician," etc.) are fictitious. Names left without such definitions are real.